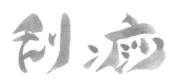

GUA SHA: A COMPLETE GUIDE TO SELF-TREATMENT

Clive Witham

Published in 2015 by Mangrove Press, UK.

ISBN: 978-0-9561507-3-8

Mangrove Press
Martello House
2 Western Road
Poole, UK

info@mangrovepress.com
www.mangrovepress.com

Disclaimer: The information in this book is given in good faith and is neither intended to diagnose any physical or mental condition nor to serve as a substitute for informed medical advice or care.

Please contact your health professional for medical advice and treatment. Neither the author nor the publisher can be held liable by any person for any loss or damage whatsoever which may arise from the use of this book or any of the information herein.

CONTENTS

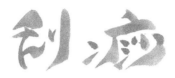

INTRODUCTION

My first experience of Gua sha was, like most people, rather unceremonious. I had stomach ache - the kind of stomach ache that seems to come out of nowhere and have you rolling about the floor, in some vain hope of relieving it.

I could have rolled myself into the car and driven to the emergency room, then squirmed around while enduring the long wait to see a doctor. I could have made it to a chemist for some pharmaceutical drug to numb the pain away. But no. My path was different.

My path to pain relief came in the form of my wife, Mutsumi, of the distinguished Japanese Ishizuka peasant lineage and mother to my children, menacingly clutching a soup spoon from the kitchen. It was clear from the take-no-prisoners glint in her eye that she would not take my whimpering protestations seriously, so I stopped rolling and adhered to her instructions, as would any patient who wants no trouble.

Mutsumi instantly put the spoon to work - not to feed me some strange healing potion but to rub my back, using a splash of oil and rhythmic movements. This silent work was interrupted now and again with her exclamations of apparent joy: "Aha! This is it. Here it comes," or "Whoa! You should see this."

But the thing is, I could not. It was all happening to my mid to lower back behind me. All I could feel was a weird sensation of some-one dragging what had been up until that moment a noodle soup spoon across my lumbar region. The spoon was no longer a spoon but a medical implement deftly wielded with dizzying speed. It was like Edward Scissorhands sculpting art from a bush, except instead of scissors, with spoons. And instead of the bush, it was my pale flesh.

It was not long before I no longer wanted to roll about the floor, and I was starting to get used to the strange sensation of what was happening behind me. At some point with me straddling a backwards-facing chair and staring down at the carpet fluff, it dawned on me that the pain was gone. Not masked like by some analgesic pharmaceutical drug, but gone. How? Why? I had no idea. All I knew was that it was spooned away, as you might remove the skin off the surface of hot milk or empty a tasty bowl of soup.

I was eventually able to coordinate a little vanity mirror in front and the full-length hall mirror behind so that I could see what that soup spoon had done to me. A sharp intake of breath later and I was transfixed. All those red marks. Drawn like thick lines of crayon on pink coloured paper. I looked spectacularly beaten, yet had felt nothing terribly unpleasant. Weird, yes; unpleasant, definitely not. In fact, I actually felt great.

It was from that moment on that I developed a profound a respect for Gua sha therapy (and kitchen utensils) and knew that I had to explore this curious technique a whole lot further.

Before I studied Oriental medicine, I used to scoff at my wife's innate knowledge of how nature can affect you. We had lived in Thailand for several years and had the ceiling fan argument frequently. It was my "Leave it on all night or I'll die of heat-stroke" versus her "You'll wake up with a cold and a stiff neck" argument. I may have won my argument every once in a while, but I sure did get a lot of colds.

My wife grew up in a time that many younger Japanese no longer know. It was before the huge technological advances that Japan is so famous for, but which have divorced many of its people from nature. You just have to look at the home she grew up in. Breaking the ice off the top of the water barrel to wash your hands in winter has been replaced by a temperature-controlled toilet seat that washes and dries you at the push of a bafflingly complex control panel. Are you in for a really big surprise if you push the wrong button!

Thankfully, I managed to instill some of this pre-technology knowledge, which was passed down from generation to generation, in my children. I did this by making radical changes in our lives. My soon-to-suffer-a-lot family was about to change countries, jobs, schools, friends, languages, and pretty much kiss civilization clean goodbye - goodbye pleasant surroundings in a suburban British bliss, and hello remote forested island in the East China Sea.

With a leap of faith on this scale, any person of sound mind would have weighed things up and assessed the risks. Only a fool would follow a dream across the world on the basis of a picture-book wedding gift. Only a dimwit would blindly jump into the unknown without a silky safety parachute - a job, a home, and so on - with which to float down gently from the skies.

In my defence I am not a 'safety parachute' kind of guy. I am the 'improvise-one-on-the-way-down-with-hopelessly-inadequate-material' kind of guy.

In the 1970s and 80s, the era when I was growing up in a London suburb, I used to watch a popular children's television programme called Blue Peter. In every show, the presenters would make useful accessories out of normal everyday materials you have in your house, such as a pen holder from toilet roll cardboard, cellotape, and glitter. That kind of thing. At the end of the show the presenters showed off their efforts, which always looked spectacular (yes, I was easily pleased back then); mine, however, was invariably awful. It would flop. No matter what it was supposed to be, it would always end up limp and gluey. And it would break at the slightest knock, too. My life parachute is more like this - cellotape and glitter rather than silk or nylon.

Despite landing well and truly in the deep end, with a home more forest than house, life on an island that consisted mostly of creepy insects and dense forest was all that I had hoped it would be, and more. This was more like the Japan of old, a place of local legends and mountain gods, where people coexisted with nature, and got from it their knowledge of life and death. People instinctively knew how to collect abalone on the seashore at just the right time; which rock pools contained octopus; the way hornets' nests can predict the coming season; in which part of the ocean schools of flying fish gathered; and countless other skills that seem to emanate from a collective pool of knowledge.

The great parachute of life has since dumped us all in the Riff Mountains in North Africa (metaphorically landing on a rather prickly cactus fruit), but none of us has forgotten our years of drawing on this vast local knowledge.

The ancient technique of Gua sha is firmly placed within this background of ancient common knowledge about nature and how it affects us. For whole swathes of the East Asia, Gua sha forms part of an innate knowledge that almost everyone seems to know but no one was ever really taught. Ideas and techniques were passed down from generation to generation within families, and reaching for a soup spoon or a coin was and often still is as common for them as opening the medicine cabinet.

This begs the question that if it is so well known and effective, why are we all not scraping our way through stomach upsets, coughs, and colds just as they do in parts of Asia? Well, we should be. The trouble with Gua sha, however, is that it is part of a medicine originating in East Asia that uses strange concepts such as 'wind' and 'qi' and 'yin' and 'yang', and although perfectly commonsensical, it sounds to some people like some kind of wacky folk remedy made up by primitive people with too much time (around two thousand years) on their hands.

There is also the added fact that it involves dragging objects across the skin, sometimes producing distinctive-looking marks and appearing more like a cruel and unusual punishment than a treatment for your health.

Introduction

This, however, is a misunderstanding. It is important not to get distracted by appearances nor by presumptions about the principles that lie behind it. Clipping your nails or shaving with a razor look horrifically painful to any onlooker not familiar with what you are doing. It is only after it has been explained and you have tried it yourself that you truly know how looks can be deceptive.

And as for Oriental medicine, with every passing year there comes more acceptance both publicly and scientifically of its merit. It is no longer the fringe medicine in the West it once was. This equally applies to Gua sha, which is being researched more and more, both in the East and in the West.

Many years after first experiencing Gua sha, and by that time also having practised it for many years clinically, I had the opportunity to witness it being used as a treatment in a hospital in Hangzhou, China. It was an eye-opening experience. As with many areas of Oriental medicine as practiced in China, there is none of the formality or sensitivity that so characterizes our approach in the West. Instead, they employ a no-nonsense approach, one that is more concerned with getting you better than how soft the treatment couch is.

This is not just confined to China - in other East Asian countries, too, there is a general cultural acceptance of discomfort. The idea behind it is that in order to improve your health you should be prepared to suffer some kind of discomfort, if such discomfort is deemed necessary. I know this because when I was in China, I would often watch patients' faces and observe their grimacing silent suffering as they were treated.

Oriental medicine and acupuncture have a word for the sensations that you feel during the initial stages of treatment: '*deqi*'. The basic concept is that without the feeling of *deqi*, the treatment will not be as effective. The exact interpretation of what constitutes *deqi* differs from place to place, but in Chinese medicine *deqi* is generally considered to be a dull ache (although there is a tendency in China to be somewhat overenthusiastic in achieving it).

Gua Sha

A recent Harvard survey of Chinese and American reactions to feeling *deqi* confirmed that Chinese participants liked this sensation, whereas the opposite rang true among American participants.[1] This in no way means that Chinese people enjoy pain more than the rest of us; it merely suggests that they have a tolerance and an expectation of discomfort in achieving health.

While my family may dispute this, I regard myself as having the grin-and-bear-it, stiff-upper-lip type of attitude to pain and discomfort. I had to admit, however, that watching the Gua sha treatment in China had me wincing once or twice in sympathy with the patient. He seemed to be bearing up fine, but that large shell implement, digging in and crunching its way down his back, was making me more than a little light-headed.

It was not only the scraping that made me feel woozy; doing the hospital rounds brought all manner of giddy wonder. This ranged from watching a patient walk out with large needles still protruding from their head like TV antennas ("It's okay. They take them out later at home.") to witnessing what essentially was an acupuncture operation (yes, an operation) to separate a knot of muscles, then being presented the giant operating needle at the end as a souvenir, as my mouth was agape the whole time.

Before we get carried away with all this pain and discomfort, however, let us start by making one thing clear: Despite being known as a technique that leads to soreness, Gua sha does not have to create discomfort in order to be effective. It is an adaptive technique that, while its roots are masculine and strong, can be just as delicate and feminine. It all depends on how and why it is used. You do not need to be like the Chinese physician bringing tears to his patient's eyes as he drags his shell-like tool across their back. There is a time and a place for this; and, indeed, Gua sha grew out of successfully treating harsh conditions like fevers and cholera. But there is also a time and a place for gentleness, awareness, and sensitivity. Think ripples on the surface rather than waves.

INTRODUCTION

Gua sha resonates deeply with this simple back-to-basics approach to healing. It is not, and never has been, reserved for experts or healers. It is part of a body of knowledge so profound and enduring that it is inconceivable that it does not belong to everyone. It was after all passed down from generation to generation and has always been more of a folk treatment to be used at home than a procedure performed in a medical centre.

Indeed, in some areas, it was quite literally seen as the people's medicine. All traditional medicine, apart from *Kos Kyal*, the Cambodian name for Gua sha, was prohibited in rural villages in Cambodia during the genocidal Khmer Rouge period from 1975–79, exactly because it was deemed to belong to the people and not the intellectual and professional classes.[2] The rest of traditional medicine was tightly controlled in what were called "factories using popular methods" and dispensed by a group of Chinese barefoot revolutionary doctors.[3] Gua sha was, however, considered base enough to be part of the revolution.

It is this idea that Gua sha is an 'informal' medicine that feels more at home in your house than in a clinic or hospital that lies behind this book. It is not designed to replace hands-on teaching if that is available to you. As in most things, it is much better to learn by doing and have someone correct you, than learn from the pages of a book. After all this is the way Gua sha was handed down through the generations. For those of you, however, without access to courses, then this book will hopefully put you on the right path to using it.

Essentially Gua sha is not the realm of expert specialists with gleaming new scrapers and painful prices. It is the realm of you and your family. Your friends. Your partners. Your neighbours.

We all collectively own it. And we owe it to ourselves to ensure that we know how to use it safely and securely.

Here's to us all.

PART 1

WHAT IS GUA SHA?

It can take a while to get your head around the idea of scraping along the skin to improve your health, but Gua sha has a long history and is widely used in East Asia. So let us start by exploring a little about its origins and how it purportedly affects the skin and body.

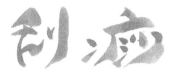

1

WHERE DOES IT COME FROM?

In order to elaborate on the origins of Gua sha, allow me to start a little closer to home. I work in Melilla, a Spanish city nestled between the Mediterranean Sea and Morocco. On a clear day, if you cross the border and climb up to the old legionnaire's fort that looms high above the city at the top of Mt.Gurugu, you can just see the jagged mountains of Tlemcen province in Algeria to the East and the Riff mountains as they head South towards the Middle Atlas. This part of the world is a mishmash of languages and cultures, but like the rest of North Africa has a long tradition of bleeding and cupping known as *Hijama*, a treatment promoted within Islam and reportedly used by the prophet Muhammad himself to maintain health.

Soon after I arrived here, I was presented with a book called 'Medicine of the Prophet' by a patient, who had explained about this 14th-century scholar's classical account of the practice of Hijama. Of course, Arabic to me is rather like algebraic equations, aesthetically beautiful but ultimately baffling. There were, however, enough ink-drawn illustrations for me to get enough of the idea to want to investigate further and dig up an English version.

It did not take very long to see the striking similarities between oriental cupping and Hijama. Both use the same technique of applying cups to suck in the skin and create a vacuum. Traditionally, a flame is dipped inside the cup to burn up the oxygen and then whisked onto the skin, where it rises inside like a balloon. You usually know that someone has had cupping treatment due to circular pink discolourations that this vacuum creates and which remain on the skin long after being treated. In both Hijama and oriental cupping, the suction cups are thought to affect a change in the balance of the body. They also both share similarities with how the body is affected by nature, with Hijama acknowledging that "diseases related to the temperament" can be caused by cold, heat, wetness, or dryness.[4] This bears some resemblance to how classical Chinese medicine sees wind, cold, heat, damp, and dryness as affecting the body's balance.

It is true however that the practice of Hijama shows marked differences from its more Eastern counterpart. This includes specific times when this treatment should be administered, notably on odd days in the second half of the lunar month (the 17th, 19th, and 21st days), ideally on a Monday, Tuesday, and Thursday. Also, it focuses on blood-letting, whereby the skin is pricked before applying the cups, which then collect the blood that comes out. This is usually termed 'wet cupping' as opposed to 'dry cupping' (without blood). And then, if we were to delve deeper into the theories of how and why cupping makes changes in the body, much deeper divisions become clear, and the cause of ill health in Hijama (blood, bilious, phlegm, and melancholic) appears closer to the Hippocratic theory of humours (blood, phlegm, yellow, and black bile) of ancient Greece than they do to Oriental medicine.

Despite these differences, however, broad similarities between the two suggest that these forms of cupping must share common ancient roots. Oriental medicine was more than a thousand years old when Islam began to spread through the Middle East in the seventh century. It makes sense, therefore, that somewhere along the ancient oriental trading routes, this knowledge had to have been shared, much like any other commodity from the East, such as silk, paper, or porcelain, or in the form of mathematics and astronomy from the West. Indeed, it was not only the Arabs but cultures as diverse as the ancient Egyptians, the Hindus, and the Greeks that used cupping and blood-letting as a medical technique.

Like cupping, Gua sha appears part of this East-West exchange. It is far from only an Asian concept and can be found in similar common traditions in other areas of the world. The ancient Greeks, for example, had the idea of 'frictioning,' which consisted of rubbing the skin with the hands, with or without oil, in order to "loosen," "harden," "increase," or "strengthen the flesh"[5].

Although limited elsewhere, what happened in East Asia is that ideas of frictioning were developed and finely tuned in the form of a specific treatment to combat certain illnesses, in particular cholera, fever, and pain. In Chinese, it got the name Gua sha (刮痧) because gua means to 'scrape' and sha refers generally to forms of disease, the disease process in the body, and also the sandy, granular, or powder-like dark spots on the skin.[6]

This technique of scraping the skin to treat and prevent illnesses became something that was passed down from generation to generation, without necessarily knowing how it works. Indeed, the understanding of many Vietnamese who use Gua sha (known as *Cao gio* in Vietnamese), for example, is purely limited to vague notions of improving circulation and removing 'wind,' and little else.[7] In reality of course there is far more to it than that, and its history is closely connected to the development of Chinese philosophy, medicine, and blood-letting and needling techniques that date back millennia.

As far as the development of Oriental medicine goes, Gua sha took very much of a backseat. It seems to have been largely ignored in classical Chinese literature. It was featured in a medical compilation by Wei Yi-Lin in the Yuan Dynasty in China called *Effective Formulas Tested by Physicians for Generations*, published in A.D.1377. In it, Wei Yi-Lin detailed the technique of scraping the surface of the neck, elbow, knee, and wrist with wet hemp until "miliary cutaneous bleeding" appears.[8]

Despite this lack of literary attention, it was widely used throughout South East Asia - not by medical practitioners but by ordinary people.[9] This, perhaps, provides the explanation for its literary absence. Ordinary people did not write books.

At the end of the 20th century, Gua sha resurged in popularity in China among a group of doctors in Taiwan. Subsequently, Professor Zhang Xiuqin developed a synthesis of the theories of microsystems, channels, and Gua sha, which she called 'Holographic Meridian Gua sha'. This led to Chinese-led research strongly focusing on how Gua sha affects the body[10], the subject of continuing research.

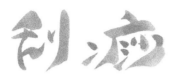

2

WHAT DOES IT DO?

As a treatment modality, Gua sha is all about the skin: what happens on it and under it. So let us now take a closer look at how Gua sha affects the skin.

Many people become aware of Gua sha after hearing about or seeing pictures like image 1.

There are understandably a lot of misunderstandings about these marks. From our previous knowledge and experience, an image like the one shown here usually suggests that something nasty or painful must have happened.

The same thing happens when you look at a photo of an acupuncture treatment. You see the needles, and your mind instantly dredges up all those old painful memories of injections, vaccinations, and blood tests. Your brain then informs you that, according to its records, you have a strong dislike of needles and sharp objects and, despite the fact that you have never seen or experienced acupuncture, it recommends that you remain in ignorance and never go and actually find out.

If you had a cough and I told you that you had a choice between spoonfuls of lemon and honey cough syrup and Gua sha (duh daah! I dramatically present you with a photo of red marks on the upper back), you are going to choose the syrup, of course. Because quite clearly the person in the photo has just undergone a nasty piece of torture, and you would much rather leave the torture to Hollywood films and stick to the syrup, which while being pretty ineffective, appears a lot more pleasant and definitely more familiar. Well, if that were your decision, you would be wrong. So, so wrong.

You would not be alone, of course. Many people react negatively to the images of red marks caused by Gua sha. Occasionally, this causes serious repercussions. One such reaction was immortalized in a 2001 film, which, believe it or not, was entitled *Gua Sha*. It featured an incident in the United States, where a doctor discovers gua sha marks on the back of the son of Chinese-American immigrants. Eventually, the whole cultural confusion is sorted out, but not before the stress of being

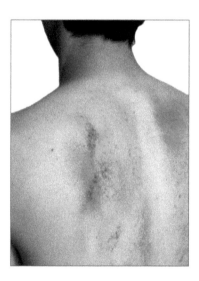

Image 1. The effects of Gua sha on the skin

accused of child abuse takes centre stage.

This reaction is not as isolated as you may think. At various times, the effects of Gua sha have been termed in emotive language, and it was not uncommon to see the words "child abuse," "trauma," "pseudo battery," and "dermabrasion" in the same sentence as Gua sha. These terms can actually be found liberally sprinkled around modern medical literature when describing the effects of Gua sha.[11]

Quite clearly, there lie some fundamental misunderstandings about Gua sha that need to be addressed.

Let us start with image 1. You may be thinking, Who on Earth would agree to let someone do that to their back? Surely grounds for a lawsuit? Well, the photo is actually of my oldest son, George, who together with son number two, Keigo, could potentially sue me for a whole bunch of reasons (dragging them all over the world since birth, refusing to upsize the TV, not owning a car, and so on), but one of them would not be Gua sha. He was (and still is) perfectly happy to tap around on his mobile while I apply Gua sha to his back to treat a cough. I just double-checked with him (a grunt I have come to learn means yes), and given the choice he would leave that cough syrup on the shelf any day of the week.

So how can I be so sure that Gua sha is not the medieval torture you might think it is?

Well, the answer to this lies in exactly what we are looking at when we see a photo like this. Has the subject (No. 1 son, George) just been beaten senseless by a brute of a man (his father, me) with a soup spoon, a piece of buffalo horn, or other random object? Is that redness considered trauma or bruising? Should we start dialling the police?

Perhaps the first hurdle is the word 'scraping'. In Gua sha the skin is 'scraped' with a smooth object. Words are loaded with preconceptions and subjective connotations, and scraping does not have the lion's share of positivity. Scraping is what Robert Shaw does in Jaws: to get the town's attention, he drags his finger nails down an old chalky blackboard. Scraping is what you do to the paintwork on your car, if your

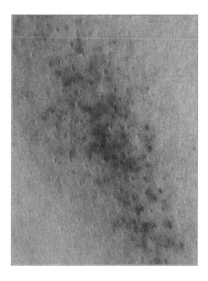

Image 2. Petechiae or Sha

parking skills are not up to scratch. Scraping is what you do to your chin, elbows, and knees, when foolishly tempted to relive your childhood on a vacant skateboard lying invitingly in your path.

The Oxford English Dictionary defines scraping as to "drag or pull a hard or sharp implement across (a surface or object) so as to remove dirt or other matter." It then goes on to give as an example the removal of the green tops from carrots and then scraping the skin off them.[12] With Gua sha, you are not doing that. You are not intending to physically remove substances from the body, as you might do to a carrot with a peeler. Clear tissue fluids and skin cells may appear outside the skin, but that is not the therapeutic aim of treatment.

The changes you are encouraging inside are actually removing the causes of ill health in a literal sense, as according to ancient oriental ideas, environmental factors such as wind, cold, and heat can enter the body through the pores of the skin and exit through sweating. In this case, there is a sense that something is actually being removed from the body and so being scraped away.

Another hurdle is what you think the image is. Despite what you may think, what you are looking at in the picture is not a bruise. According to Black's Medical Dictionary, which has propped up the other books on my bookshelf for many years - so much so that I had to blow the dust off like a scene of an old movie - bruises are "contusions" that "result from injuries to the deeper layers of skin or underlying tissues, with variable bleeding, but without open wounds."[13] A contusion is caused by a blow or strike and causes a localized deep injury.

It might look like it to you, but image 2 is not showing an injury - nothing has struck the body to cause damage. Instead, the redness that you can see is something known as *petechiae* (pe-tee-kiya). The same dusty dictionary can shed light on this. Petechiae are "small red macules due to haemorrhage in the skin." (A macule, by the way, is a patch of skin that has changed colour). The patch is actually made up of pin-point dots up to one millimetre in diameter, and are often clustered together so that they appear larger.

Petechiae appear when the muscle fibres and connective tissue underneath are pressed but the skin remains unbroken. If this were a bruise, blood from the ruptured small blood vessels close to the surface of the skin (capillaries) would escape by leaking out under the skin. But in Gua sha, the capillaries remain unbroken. The leakage is from what is known as the capillary bed of surface tissue.[14] Unable to leave the body, this blood then gets trapped in the extravascular space under the skin and forms red or purple dots.

The ancient Chinese did not have a modern understanding of the formation of petechiae, instead the redness on the skin was called *sha* and as you will find out in the next section, represented a fundamental change in what is happening inside the body.

So Gua sha therapy is not trauma. It is not a bruise. It is not abuse. It is a very effective manual treatment to help the body heal itself. And remember that it does not have to draw petechiae to the surface to be effective. It all depends on the goal of treatment. Which of course leads us on to another very important question. How exactly does it work?

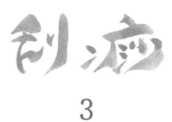

3

HOW DOES IT WORK?

I once had the opportunity to work as a professional wood crafts-man in Japan, and although I remained very much the green apprentice, my skilled employers used to produce some exquisite works from some of the finest wood in the world. Each piece was made from Yakusugi, a unique species of Japanese cedar, and carved from fallen trees that were over a thousand years old. Just to work with this wood was a privilege. Every layer revealed a different pattern, and, therefore, a different story, in the life of these ancient trees.

If I were to put a beautifully carved piece of Yakusugi on the table in front of you, you would probably pick it up and admire the crafts-manship. You might comment on the appearance of the figure. How it is weighted at the bottom. How you could use it for all kinds of useful things - a paperweight, a decorative ornament, an ink stamp. You would definitely smell it, and draw in the sweet scent of ageing sugi. You might even admire the lifelike quality of the carved face, and how the natural oil of the Yakusugi wood gives it its distinctive character and colour. In short, you would appreciate it for the art that it is, snap it up, and have it adorn the mantelpiece above your fireplace for years to come.

The trouble is that, for all the skill and artistry behind it, what you just bought and appreciated is not what it seems.

Yes, it is a beautifully carved piece, but you could never really understand what it is and why it was so lovingly made unless you could actually see it sitting on the chess board it was made for, surrounded by the other similarly carved pieces. Your carving is actually a chess piece and part of something much bigger, but you would only know this if you saw the chequered board. And only if you understood the game of chess could you really appreciate where this piece fits in and how, far from being static, it moves so gracefully across the board.

Similarly, if I presented you with a Gua sha treatment without placing it in the healing context in which it was formed, then it is like a chess piece without a board - a major part of it would be missing. As much as some people might want to, you cannot divorce an idea from its origins. For some, the talk of energy medicine, of the interaction of environmental factors like wind and heat and damp, of a system of channels in the body, may sound splendidly unscientific. But then again, similar reservations were expressed when the West first heard about the strange Eastern practice of putting needles in your skin. Every year brings more scientifically verified proof that acupuncture works. Exactly how is an ongoing scientific debate, but it is no longer a weird fringe medicine; on the contrary, it is now very much mainstream.

So to put Gua sha into its context, let us first look at "the chess board" of which it is part:

Qi and blood

Oriental medicine works with the concept that *qi* (chee) or *ki* (kee) flows around the body as water does in rivers and streams. This *qi* is often misinterpreted as 'energy' in English, as there is no fit translation for it; however, it should more correctly be viewed as a combination of 'energetic phenomena' in the body, much like we see nerve impulses, the transfer of signals between cells, or the metabolic transformation of food as energetic processes. *Qi* is not energy, but it is energetic.

How does it work?

It is this *qi* that powers and protects the body and is involved in anything we do, from static breathing to running along the street. It works in combination with blood, which among other functions nourishes the muscles and tendons, moisturizes the skin, and lubricates joints and cavities.

If the flow of blood and *qi* is weak, there is a tendency for it to accumulate and collect in pools. We only have to look at the natural world to see how pools of standing water behave. The lack of movement in a stream or river means that the water becomes stagnant. It becomes easily clogged up with all sorts of dense materials and organisms, such as algae, anaerobic bacteria, and biofilm. It is a similar (but less green and slimy) process when blood and *qi* are blocked in the body. The lack of movement creates stagnation, which usually results in discomfort and pain.

The general idea is that using Gua sha near the area of pain will release the local area of stagnation, thereby improving the flow of blood and *qi*. When this flow improves, the discomfort is then decreased.

But in order to grasp the full extent of this idea of flowing *qi* and blood, you need to be aware of the fact that Oriental medicine conceives of these 'rivers' of *qi* as running along distinct channels up and down the body in what are known as channels or meridians.

The presence of these channels of *qi* means that scraping on a completely different body part to the one where you may feel discomfort can relieve that same discomfort. Gua sha applied to a particular channel has an effect on the whole channel, not just that part, and will improve the flow throughout, not just in that area. This is rather like what a plumber might do when flushing out the water pipes of a house. It is not necessary to work directly on the obstructed area in order to clear it. Removal of the blockage is achieved by working on the whole piping system and opening up all the faucets in the house.

GUA SHA

THE CHANNEL SYSTEM

Let us now look a little closer at the body's energetic plumbing. One of the main tenets of Oriental medicine is that the body functions through a network of channels, or meridians, and branches carrying and distributing vital *qi* and blood. It is much like the more familiar idea of how oxygen and blood are transported through arteries, veins, and capillaries, but with one main difference: while you can open up the body and see the network of blood vessels, you cannot do the same with the channels carrying *qi*. This does not mean, of course, that they are not there. They are not just the figment of several thousand years' worth of medical practitioners' imaginations or wishful thinking. It is just that instead of being a separate physical entity, they exist at a more subtle level of the body's connective tissue and muscle mass.

It is thought that these *qi* channels, or meridians, follow natural tissue planes between muscles, or between muscles and bones or tendons. Manipulation at areas where these planes converge is believed to send mechanical signals to connective tissue cells by converting them into chemical or electrical signals, a process known as mechanotransduction.[15]

Let's take a common trauma in the leg as an example. I once trained to run the London marathon, but just at the key moment in training, a month before the race, when I was supposed to reach the peak of physical fitness, I had the foolish idea of running across wet grass, slid on a patch of mud, and twisted my ankle. It swelled up immediately and even the simplest movement was painful for weeks to come. Twisting an ankle, I am sure, is a familiar situation for many people. If all goes well, with rest and painkillers, you can start to move again and with more time, the pain goes away, movement returns, and soon the incident is all but forgotten. In my case, you end up half-killing yourself in the marathon the following year instead.

Sometimes, however, while the injury will heal just fine, there is a lingering pain or ache that never really goes away. Investigations and tests all come back clear, and there is nothing demonstrably wrong. But you still have pain. It is a surprisingly common scenario, and in some cases even leads to psychological evaluations to explain the sufferers' feelings of pain ("But it's not all in my head!").

The lingering pain or ache is usually connected to the fact that it was not only your body tissue, blood vessels, or muscle or ligament fibres that were damaged, but the channel system. Let us return to my swollen blue ankle to see how.

It was the outside of the ankle that had taken the brunt of the damage and was spectacularly outsized. Two channels run over this area: the Gall bladder and the Bladder channels. Both of them start up at the head, go down the body and end at the nail beds in the toes. The swelling was an obstruction preventing these channels from completing their circuit to the toes.

The rest of me being fit and healthy, I was able to regularly treat these channels to ensure that all traces of the obstruction was gone. I did this with something that sounds like a ninja weapon, the seven star hammer. In fact, like Gua sha, the hammer looks rather scary at first glance with seven needles protruding out of a slender plastic base. But once you get over what it looks like, it is truly a marvellous tool and with a little regular tapping, Gua sha, and using needles in the main acupuncture points in the body that affected the channels of that particular area, the swollen obstruction was history.

Knowledge of where these channels run in combination with basic anatomy can therefore prove very useful in treating and preventing ill health.

The main channels are illustrated here to give you a rough idea about their trajectories. They are colour coded according to their traditional correspondence with the five elements. The lighter colours are the yin channels, which are mainly located on the interior or front of the body, and the darker colours are the yang channels, mainly located on the exterior or the back.

DIRECTIONS OF MAIN CHANNELS

Like blood vessels, the channels are thought to have a directional flow either up or down the body and limbs.

ARM CHANNELS

These are commonly referred to as the arm channels, but they either originate from the chest or continue up to the face and head. They are used frequently for therapeutic purposes as, being on the arm, they are very accessible, especially when treating yourself, and also the fact that they contain many potent body points.

Yang Channels (Up)

These are known as yang channels and go from the nail points of the hands to the head:

- △ Large intestine channel (dark grey) - associated with the front of the head, nose, and mouth.
- △ Triple burner channel (dark purple) - associated with the side of the head, ears, ribs, and stomach area.
- △ Small intestine channel (dark red) - associated with the back of the head, shoulder, and ears.

All of these channels are connected to the treatment of fevers.

Yin Channels (Down)

These are known as yin channels and go from the chest to the nail points of the hands:

- △ Lung channel (light grey) - associated with the respiratory system.
- △ Pericardium channel (light purple) - associated with heart, stomach, and mental issues.
- △ Heart channel (light red) - associated with the heart and

mental issues.

All of these channels are associated with problems related to the chest area.

LEG CHANNELS

These are commonly referred to as the leg channels, but most of them travel across the body and either begin or end in the chest or head. Like the arm channels, the legs often contain powerful points that can be used to facilitate changes in the body and are very accessible to treat.

Yin Channels (Up)

These are known as yin channels and flow from the nail points of the feet to the chest:

- △ Spleen channel (yellow) - associated with problems in the stomach and spleen.
- △ Kidney channel (light blue) - associated with respiratory and kidney issues.
- △ Liver channel (light green) - associated with the liver.

All of these channels are connected to the treatment of gynaecological problems.

Yang Channels (Down)

These are called yang channels and go from the head to the nail points of the feet:

- △ Stomach channel (orange) - associated with the front of the head, mouth, stomach, and intestines.
- △ Bladder channel (dark blue) - associated with the back, back of the head, waist, and eyes.

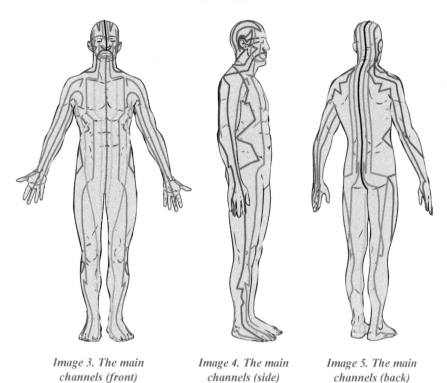

| *Image 3. The main channels (front)* | *Image 4. The main channels (side)* | *Image 5. The main channels (back)* |

△ Gall bladder channel (dark green) - associated with the side of the head, ears, and eyes.

EXTRA CHANNELS

These channels flow up the front and back of the body, both ending at the mouth area:

Yin Channels (Up)

△ Ren or Conception channel (light brown) regulates all the yin channels and is traditionally associated with gynaecological issues.

Yang Channels (Down)

△ Du or Governing channel (black) regulates all the yang channels. It is traditionally related to the functions of the brain, marrow, and kidneys.

These 14 channels form part of the channel system which, like the human body, is infinitely complicated, with a whole host of branches connecting channels, extra channels and skin regions. All play a role in helping us understand how the body functions, but for the purposes of helping us understand the workings of Gua sha, the obvious extension to the channel system to pay attention to is the theory of working with the cutaneous regions.

Cutaneous regions

In Oriental medicine theory, the channels are viewed as flowing beneath the skin, but they also have a direct connection with it. The cutaneous regions refer to areas where *qi* and blood contained in the channels are transferred to the skin. This idea is so old that it was found in excavated scrolls from the third century BCE, one of which was a medical classic called Plain Questions.[16] It describes how distinct surface areas in the body are ruled by the 12 main internal channels.

Astonishingly, these ancient ideas are just as relevant today as they were thousands of years ago, and especially relevant to the practice of Gua sha. This is because these cutaneous areas provide us with the theoretical foundation for the concept that natural environmental phenomena can pass through the skin and sink ever deeper into the body to affect the balance of health. The idea that we are working with here is that the skin is the first stage of disease.

For example, when a pathogen like cold enters the body, it first passes through the skin to the superficial channels (known technically as the 'minute collaterals' and 'sinew channels'), then to the main channels (the 'luo-connecting' and 'primary channels'), and then the deep

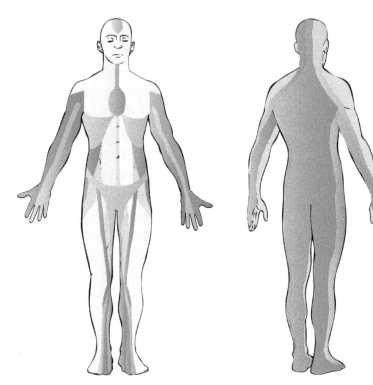

*Image 6. The cutaneous
regions (front)*   *Image 7. The cutaneous
regions (back)*

channels (the 'extraordinary channels' and 'deep pathways'). In this way,
cold can gradually move deeper into the body. It becomes more prob-
lematic for your health the further it gets through this layered channel
system. Cold is just one of several external factors that are thought
to penetrate through the body and cause illness. The others are heat,
damp, wind, and dryness.

In the case of a common cold virus, typical symptoms include a
runny nose, sneezing, sore throat, a stiff neck, and a headache, which
according to Oriental medicine theory, are caused by the superficial

penetration of wind and cold into the body.

At the beginning stage, the wind and cold are not very deep and can be expelled with the appropriate treatment, normally one that involves or mimics the action of sweating.

If the condition is left without treatment, there exists the possibility that the wind and cold will penetrate deeper into the body and affect the lungs, such as with a prolonged cough and the buildup of phlegm. It can then go even deeper and start to affect other organs and channels. The disruption can easily lead to stagnation, and the cold can then transform into heat. So what started off as a few sniffles can end with a strong health imbalance.

This whole external-internal process also works to disturb health in the opposite direction, and in Oriental medicine, it is believed that signs and symptoms of internal organ and channel imbalances can manifest directly on the skin. This means that sensations, marks, lesions, and discolourations on the skin do not have to be localized skin issues but part of a messaging system whereby the body is signalling an internal imbalance on the exterior of the body. Obvious examples of this are the classical descriptions that a blue-green skin colour is indicative of pain, red skin suggests heat, and white skin points to weakness and cold.

As this connection between the skin and the channels and organs was clearly established within the very foundations of channel theory all those years ago, Oriental medicine has a built-in explanation of how you can treat the skin area and have a profound therapeutic effect much deeper in the body.

The theory of cutaneous regions divides the skin surface area into six distinct zones of influence, each related to two primary channels - one from the arms and one from the legs (see images 6 and 7).

△ TAIYANG or supreme yang – Small intestine (on the arm) and Bladder (on the leg)

△ SHAOYANG or lesser yang – Triple burner (on the arm) and Gall bladder (on the leg)

△ YANGMING or yang brightness – Large intestine (on the arm) and Stomach (on the leg)

△ TAIYIN or supreme yin – Lung (on the arm) and Spleen (on the leg)

△ JUEYIN or absolute yin – Pericardium (on the arm) and Liver (on the leg)

△ SHAOYIN or lesser yin – Heart (on the arm) and Kidney (on the leg)

So now that we have seen the chessboard and have had a short introduction in the game of chess, let us now see how the actual piece itself, Gua sha, works.

There are essentially two main ways Gua sha works as a treatment: one is to get things moving again, and the other is to expel unwanted intrusion of natural phenomena.

Gua sha clears qi and blood stagnation

In China, a phrase that is often used to explain how Gua sha works is that it is 'dredging the channels.' If I told you this without your knowing a little about the underlying theories of Oriental medicine, you might understandably be looking for the emergency exit signs so that you slip away quietly. It does not sound particularly scientific, nor indeed medical. In fact, you might think that I am referring to removing the leaves from the gutters rather than to a procedure for your health.

Nevertheless, if we take into account that channels can be demonstrated as natural planes of connective tissue, and that connective tissue is actually a sensitive signalling system, it makes sense to do a little spring cleaning along these channels. If there is a blockage causing a problem, you unblock it. As you will recall, channels are thought to have a directional flow of blood and *qi*, so 'dredging,' or strongly clearing them, will improve the flow and prevent them from stagnating.

Pain, for example, is thought to be essentially a blood or *qi* obstruction. The traditional idea is that the smooth flow of blood and *qi* has been blocked, which causes pressure to build up from behind and then leads to symptomatic messages to draw your attention to it. It could be obstructed due to a weakness in *qi* or blood, in that it is not plentiful or strong enough to flow smoothly, or it could be that the state of the rest of the body has placed obstacles in its path, such as how the body reacts with stress and strong emotional disturbances like frustration and anger.

Either way, localized clearing of stagnation will benefit the whole body by improving the blood flow but also in helping any underlying weakness by encouraging the body to produce blood.

GUA SHA EXPELS ENVIRONMENTAL FACTORS

Oriental medicine developed ideas thousands of years ago that help explain the complex processes of how the body becomes ill through environmental phenomena. Rather than viewing humans as distinct from nature, Oriental medicine theory views man as intrinsically linked to nature, in a constant daily interaction with the natural environment around us, no matter where we are.

For example, you might believe that your stiff neck is due to the position you slept in last night, but in Oriental medicine, it would be considered whether perhaps sitting close to the air conditioner the day before had caused wind to invade the superficial channels of the body and that this was the source of the neck pain.

Or that stubborn backache that just will not go away - the one that your doctor thinks might be related to a weak vertebral disc - it could very well be connected to getting soaked in the rain and the cold and damp seeping through to your particular weak point, the lower back.

Or your barking expectorant cough, which does not respond well to cough remedies, perhaps it could be heat and phlegm obstructing your lungs because you did not take care of yourself the last time you caught a cold.

It may sound strange, but if we take into account that there is more to health than the reductionist confines of modern medicine, and we embrace the fact that we are a product of the environment that we live in, then these explanations may not sound so strange.

As mentioned above in the cutaneous region section, cold, heat, wind, and damp pass through different stages in the body. If still confined to an exterior stage, they can be expelled and prevented from penetrating any farther by 'releasing the exterior' and inducing sweating via Gua sha, with the aim of expelling the environmental factor through the open pores along with the sweat. Sweating also helps expel heat, which often takes the form of a fever, thereby providing a vent that allows the body to cool.

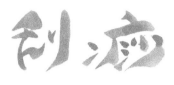

4

WHO IS IT FOR?

While Gua sha is a general effective treatment, there are some conditions and some body areas which require caution. So let us start with these - who and where it is not for.

Do not use Gua sha techniques on yourself if you have the following:

△ blood clotting limitations (e.g. you are a haemophiliac or on anticoagulant medication)
△ weak, thin skin (e.g. you are elderly or on steroids)
△ on your abdomen or lower back area if you are pregnant

Do not use Gua sha techniques on the following areas:

△ directly over an area of recent trauma
△ over broken or ulcerated skin
△ over varicose veins or other enlarged blood vessels
△ over an area with oedema (an excessive buildup of fluid in body tissue)

△ over a thrombosis (a clot in a blood vessel), an aneurysm (a bulge in a blood vessel), or advanced arteriosclerosis (a thickening of the arteries).[17]

WHO IT IS FOR?

There is a mistaken belief that Gua sha is only for something. If you have sore shoulders, you need Gua sha. If you have a bad back, you need Gua sha. If you have a cold, you need Gua sha. But Gua sha is much more than treating an ailment. Regular Gua sha used along the lines shown in this book, has a preventative and balancing quality which means that you can actually help prevent the ailment from appearing in the first place.

As regards imbalances, the underlying idea in Gua sha is one of moving stagnation and improving circulation, which means that indications of Gua sha are wide and varied. Any situation in which there may be stagnation, especially over a period of time, as in the case of chronic health conditions, means that Gua sha may help.

CHRONIC CONDITIONS

If a condition is chronic, it is persistent and usually interferes with how you live your life. Chronic conditions include arthritis, diabetes, asthma, high blood pressure, obesity, and heart disease and are increasingly common all over the world. A large European study of how chronic pain affects people found that pain of moderate-to-severe intensity occurred in 19 percent of the adults surveyed and seriously affected the quality of their social and working lives.[18]

Chronic conditions normally involve some kind of obstruction in the flow of blood and *qi*, either as part of the problem or alongside it.

Chronic lower back pain, for example, can be debilitating, as even simple body movements can cause extreme discomfort. There are many possible causes of back pain, from trauma to the spine to cold and damp settling into the tissues, but the sheer fact that movement is restricted will encourage an obstruction of the free movement of blood and nutritive *qi*. So whether or not the back problem is caused by an obstruction, it will develop one in time.

Many people who suffer pain or discomfort do so in connection with the movement (or lack of movement) of their joints. This could be chronic, as with some types of arthritis, or acute, as with a sports injury. Especially in the case of chronic joint pain, such as arthritis, few treatment options are available in modern allopathic medicine; what does exist usually involves pharmaceutically masking the pain and little else. In Oriental medicine, however, this condition is considered to be one of stagnation, and the moving and anti-inflammatory action of Gua sha can help in many cases.

Another example is chronic headaches. In Oriental medical practice, the cause of the headache is rarely found to be actually located in the head; instead, the pain in the head is usually symptomatic of an issue elsewhere in the body. Commonly, when headaches are chronic, the whole neck and shoulder area has accumulated a level of obstruction that has knotted or contracted the muscles, thereby preventing blood and *qi* from rising smoothly into the head.

In most cases of chronic pain like these, Gua sha can be helpful, as it can help to resolve the stagnation in the body or improve the flow around the obstruction.

ACUTE CONDITIONS

The introduction to this book about my first experience with Gua sha should tell you that the pain does not have to be chronic to benefit from using this ancient technique. In fact, the speed at which an acute condition can be resolved is one of the most astonishing features of the practice of Gua sha. Far from being a supporting therapy, Gua sha has traditionally been used as a first-stage treatment for a whole host of ailments. It was historically seen as form of home first aid to stop illnesses in their tracks, or to prevent their appearance in the first place. It was, after all, originally developed as a first-stage counteractive treatment for acute conditions such as fevers and cholera.[19]

Recent studies have also looked at the effectiveness of Gua sha in treating acute conditions such as respiratory infections, hepatitis, conjunctivitis, pharyngitis, sinusitis, bronchitis, pneumonia, and influenza.[20] With acute conditions like these, where the symptoms appear quickly and the problem is normally short-lived yet potentially severe, there is a greater likelihood that sha will appear on the skin and that it will be a deeper colour.

If you catch a cold, for example, the body spends the initial stage fighting it off. You may get symptoms like sneezing, a sore throat, a headache, and chills or fever. This is part of your immune response - your body's immune system is attempting to combat the virus with white blood cells known as T and B lymphocytes. In Oriental medicine terms, it is a similar process, except instead of a virus, a cold is seen as wind, and the body attempts to repel this wind using its superficial layer of defensive *qi*.

Applying Gua sha to the upper back helps to promote this expulsion of wind (or relieve the body of the virus) by opening the pores and mimicking the action of sweating. This process, as was explained in the previous section, is known as 'releasing the exterior' and is used as a way to expel wind, cold, heat, and any other environmental factor from the body. The upper back is particularly affected, as the invasion of wind is associated with the lungs and the respiratory system.

Changeable Symptoms

Sometimes, if you have a pain or ache you massage it and it feels better for a while, but then it returns again later. Other aches and pains come and go, seemingly at random, although that is rarely the case. There is always a connection; it is just that you do not always know it. It may be the weather, your recent activity, your posture, the time of day, or a whole host of other factors. What is actually going on is often connected to the localized stagnation of blood and *qi* that is temporarily improved by manipulation of tissues, as in massage, for example. When the mobilization of blood and *qi* that accompanies manipulation of the body has worn off, stagnation resumes.

Deep-seated stagnation in the body is one of the prime indicators that Gua sha treatment is needed in order to bring the stagnation to the surface and resolve the condition. What this really means in therapeutic terms is that the area of the body treated should be expanded beyond the affected area. For example, say that you have a pain in your knee joint that comes and goes and, despite all your best efforts, keeps returning. Doing Gua sha near the knee is often not enough. You have to think in terms of the body as a whole, not just the knee. It is usually necessary to do Gua sha farther along the leg and stroke along the channels that pass over the knee area. It might also be appropriate to treat the back and the same areas on the other leg.

PART 2

HOW DO YOU DO GUA SHA?

Gua sha involves far more than just rubbing a flat object across the skin. You need to take into account the tool, the skin friction, posture, pressure, stoke technique, direction, and a whole host of other factors that can influence what you do and the results that it brings.

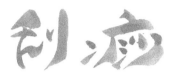

5

WHAT TOOLS DO YOU NEED?

Before looking at the techniques and procedures used in a Gua sha treatment, you need to make sure you are using appropriate equipment.

TOOLS

The basic equipment needed to perform Gua sha is actually very simple. You need to hold a smooth rounded object, which can take a variety of forms, to move over the skin. This object, in turn, needs something between it and your skin to reduce any friction and avoid discomfort. Sometimes this takes the form of thin material, such as your clothes, but more often it is a type of lubricant, such as oils or creams.

All kinds of tools can be used in Gua sha therapy. Traditionally, materials like flax, sandalwood, or clam shell were used, but the general rule is whatever you use, it must have a rounded edge so that it does not damage the skin. It should not be too sharp nor should it be too blunt, as either could cause discomfort.

Gua Sha

The instrument of choice in many East Asian countries has traditionally been a worn-down coin, hence Gua sha is sometimes known as "coining." This, however, is probably not the most comfortable of tools, and with the other options available, would not be your first choice.

Homemade tools

You do not have to scroll through website stores on the internet to find that special Gua sha tool made from some rare precious stone and sporting an equally precious price tag. You can actually start, as people have done since ancient times, with the objects that might be lying around your home, which can be adapted to the practice of Gua sha.

The two most common are the following:

Chinese soup spoon

Most people either have, or can easily get hold of, Chinese soup spoons. They are usually made from porcelain and have a flat bottom in order not to spill your soup. The edge of the spoon is much smoother than the metallic spoons sitting in the cutlery draw and when held at an angle to the skin should glide across it without it being uncomfortable. Be aware that, like people, not all Chinese soup spoons are alike, so ensure that the sides are smooth and rounded before use.

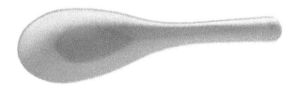

Image 8. Chinese Soup Spoon

What tools do you need?

Lid or cap

The type of covered metallic lid often found on a jar of jam or marmalade with a smooth rounded edge can be used for Gua sha. It must, of course, be a lid that is no longer used, and it has the added benefit of being both cheap and disposable, avoiding any dangers of cross-contamination (see Is IT SAFE? on page 71 for more on this).

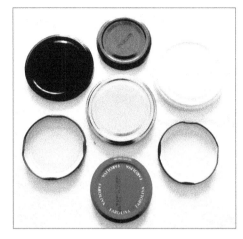

Image 9. Jar lids

SPECIALLY PRODUCED TOOLS

Some people buy a specially made tool for Gua sha. These can easily be found online or in Chinese medicine shops. The benefits of these, as they are designed especially for Gua sha therapy, are that they are moulded into convenient shapes to treat different body parts.

The most common shapes for specifically designed Gua sha tools are fish or duck feet, rectangles, and horn shapes but there seems to be an almost unlimited variation on these, ranging from cheap and simple to jaw-droppingly expensive. These tools can usually be found made from similar materials.

Buffalo Horn Tool

The most common tool produced in East Asia is buffalo horn, which has a smooth, polished appearance and is made up of dense layers of fibres that give it a very hard and durable surface. It is often used in Gua sha because of this, but also as it has the benefit of being flatter and more rectangular than the horns of cattle, and so can be made into more versatile shapes. The problem with some types of buffalo horn, however, is that they bend and eventually become brittle if left wet or

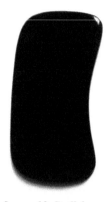

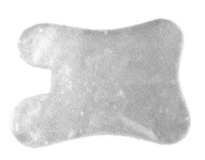

Image 10. Buffalo Horn tool

Image 11. Jade tool

immersed in water for too long.

Jade Tool

Various stones and minerals are shaped especially for Gua sha, the most common of which is probably jade. In East Asia, jade has always been a prized precious stone, with qualities of beauty, purity, and durability. It is also thought to have a healing, cooling quality. The main problem with jade, however, is that it can break easily if dropped on a hard surface.

Other Tools

Other materials that you may come across include obsidian (a type of volcanic glass), basalt stone, plastic, and metal. Metal tools are often associated with techniques in physiotherapy known as Grastan Technique and Augmented Soft Tissue Mobilization (ASTYM), which are essentially modern, shiny, and rather expensive adaptations of Gua sha - prime examples of the chess piece without the board.

What tools do you need?

Lubricants

It is commonly understood that in order to enjoy the therapeutic effects of Gua sha, you have to scrape directly on the skin with lubricant. There are, however, other ways of applying Gua sha.

Without any Lubrication

Gua sha can be used to scrape over light clothing. This was traditionally done when using Gua sha with children and older, weaker people but, in fact, it can used on anyone.

Take as an example the first signs of a cold. One rapid remedy is to scrape down the forearm from the elbow crease to the wrist following the Lung channel. Divide this area into three, and stroke three times in each third until you reach the wrist, repeating the sequence several times. Skin lubrication is not always available or convenient, but this simple technique is something that can be done effectively through your clothes (although best with no more than one layer of material).

Other areas of the body can be treated in a similar way. At the end of a stressful day, you may feel the weight of that stress tensing up your shoulder and neck muscles. Simply scraping through your clothes in this area will help to alleviate some of the tension.

With lubrication

Any direct scraping on the skin needs a lubricant, so as not to damage the skin or cause pain. Traditionally, oil or water were used, but you can buy all sorts of scraping oils and creams in Chinese supermarkets, herbal suppliers, or websites online. These are normally pre-blended concoctions of oils and herbs that are specifically aimed at massage or Gua sha treatments. But like with the tools, you can start with what you already have at home.

Homemade

Soap and Water

Why complicate things? When doing Gua sha treatment on yourself, an obvious place to practise it is in the bath or shower. In this way,
all you need is soap as the lubricant and water to wash it off.

Cooking Oils

Common vegetable oils that you might have in the kitchen provide
a good consistency on the skin for Gua sha treatment. Oils like almond,
safflower, sunflower, avocado, grapeseed, olive, and sesame are often
used as a base oil in massage therapy, and therefore can also be applied
with Gua sha.

Specially made lubricants

Massage and Essential Oils

Gua sha works on the skin surface, so any kind of blended oil
aimed at massage can be used in Gua sha.

Petroleum-based Products

You may be familiar with using Vaseline, or petroleum jelly, to
prevent chaffing (cyclers and joggers, especially), to moisten your lips,
or to stop chapped hands, but it serves just as well as a smooth lubricant
for Gua sha. The same is true of other petroleum-based products, such
as vapour rub. Vapour rub mixes petrolatum with camphor, turpentine,
menthol, eucalyptus, and globules leaf oil. Known by many as a de-

congestant to ease breathing, the additional oils in the mixture give it a warming and moving quality for blood and *qi*, which are very useful in Gua sha.

Blended Lubricants

Commercial lubricants for use in Gua sha are readily available. These usually contain oils and herbs with strong moving and damp-resolving properties in order to improve the circulation of blood and *qi*. They are not usually recommended for use during pregnancy or with young children, and they should not be used in excess.

The most commonly available include the following:

- △ GUASHAYOU: A safflower and camphor oil concoction with added herbs to promote blood circulation, eliminate chills, and relax muscles.
- △ PO SUM: A medicated oil with a peppermint oil and camelia oil base and added herbs (including dragon's blood) to move the blood.
- △ WHITE FLOWER OIL: A mixture of wintergreen, menthol, camphor, eucalyptus, and lavender oils.
- △ RED FLOWER OIL: A mixture of wintergreen, cinnamon leaf, clove, and citronella oils
  (Note: both of the above oil blends are designed to have a soothing and warming effect on the body by regulating and calming the liver, and therefore relaxing and helping the body circulate blood and *qi*.)
- △ TIGER BALM (RED/WHITE): A combination of camphor oil, cajuput and clove oil, menthol, and herbs in a petroleum jelly base.
- △ BEE BRAND OIL (MINYAK GOSOK): An old Indonesian collection of heating herbs and oils, including coconut, camphor, menthol, clove, lemongrass, ginger, and garlic. It is sold

as a topical analgesic and normally used on aching muscles
and joints to improve circulation.

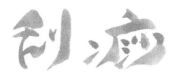

6

HOW DO YOU USE THE TOOLS?

PREPARE YOUR MINDSET

It is a good thing to be in the right frame of mind to practise Gua sha. If your mind is elsewhere, full of worries and preoccupations, you will not be able to focus on what you are doing, and instead of being a healing experience, the treatment then becomes nothing more than a mechanical scraping action.

For several years, I practised Qi gong, an ancient Chinese method of movement, breathing, and exercise similar to Tai chi. Try as I may, I was always notoriously bad at it. Instead of letting my mind go free and allowing the gentle flowing movements to interact with the balance of my *qi*, I pondered about the dinner I would have after the class and what movie to watch after that. It was the same with karate. I actually broke a bone in my foot during grading at the Budokan in Tokyo and then secretly hid the fact (and the shame) as I knelt on the floor for the next three agonizing hours. One piece of wood. Fine. Two. Okay. But focusing enough *qi* in my flying foot to smash three. They had the wrong guy.

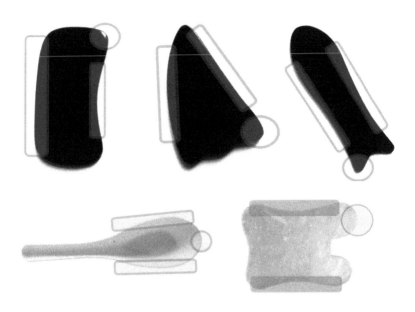

Image 12-16. Sides and corners of tools

I have since come to realize that meditative states come in many shapes and forms - from meditation, yoga, and martial arts to watching the sun set, doing the washing up, and running (I was as peaceful as a guru when I did marathon training). You do not have to be in the corner chanting a mantra (although feel free to do so), but you do need to focus on what you are doing, relax your shoulders, clear your mind, and let the repetitive motions form a more meditative state. You are more likely to respond to the way your body is reacting to the Gua sha tool if you are calm and relaxed.

Your hold on the tool should be firm but not tight. Your wrist and elbow joints should be loose, and the stroking movement should come from the elbow or shoulder. Think of the tool as an extension of your arm, and move accordingly.

How do you use the tools?

Apply the lubricant

Apply sufficient lubricant directly to the skin and not to the tool.

It is important not to over- or under-lubricate. Too much and the lack of friction dulls the therapeutic effect of Gua sha; too little and the dragging action of the tool becomes painful.

Tool techniques

One person's specialised jade scraping tool is another person's Chinese soup spoon, and we do not all have access to the same tools. The following Gua sha techniques, therefore, are based on using different types of tool to carry out the treatment.

Whichever tool you use, the only proviso is to be sure that the sides have smooth, rounded edges and the corner has a narrower rounded edge (for the purposes of this book, the longer flatter part of the tool is the 'side,' and the more rounded narrower end is the 'corner.') Images 12-16 indicate the location of these areas on commonly available Gua sha tools. Exactly how you use each part of the tool depends on your body shape and which body part is being treated.

Stroke techniques

I. Wide stroke

Use the side part of the Gua sha tool to press and stroke (at the same time) with the tool. Each stroke should be measured, firm, have sufficient pressure, and be at an angle consistent with the type of treatment you are giving (tonifying or purging - see Is it the same for everyone? on page 66 for more details).

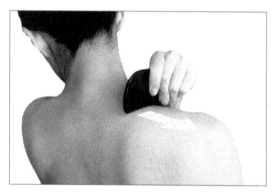

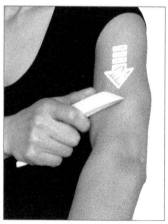

Images 17-18. Wide stroke

II. Narrow stroke

This stroke is similar to side stroke. The difference is that you use the rounded end of the tool to stroke instead of the longer side, which means that the surface area of the skin treated is much narrower and the effect is therefore more focused.

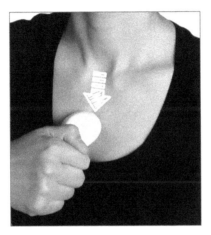

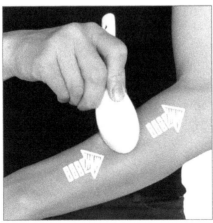

Images 19-20. Narrow stroke

III. Vibrate

Use the rounded end of the tool, as you would in narrow stroke, but instead, use a short vigorous back and forth stroking action on one fixed point while simultaneously pressing down the tool slightly.

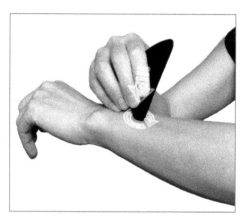

NOTE: If you are using this technique on the head, use the side of the tool rather than the corner.

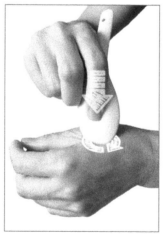

Images 21-22. Vibrate

IV. Press

Use the rounded corner of the tool to press on a fixed point. Hold the tool in place for 5–10 seconds.

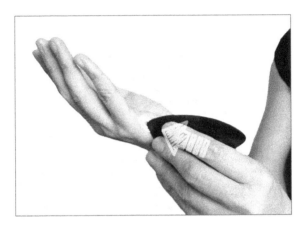

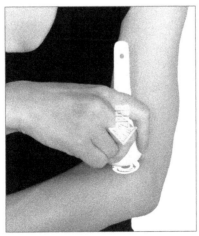

Images 23-24. Press

V. Circle

Using the rounded corner of the tool and applying light pressure only, slowly move forwards using a circular motion. The tool itself stays on one fixed point on the skin, while the combined circular movement

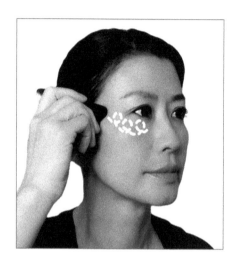

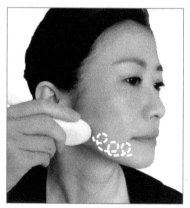

Images 25-26. Circle

of the arm, wrist, and tool creates a similar movement in the tissues under the skin. Then move your arm smoothly to another fixed point, and repeat the circular motion.

STROKE LENGTH

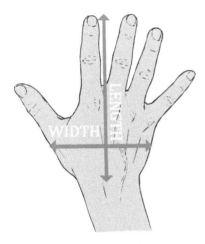

Image 27. Stroke length

For wide stroke and narrow stroke, the length of each stroke should be uniform. This depends on the body part, but in general each stroke should be somewhere between the width and length of your hand.

On the face and head, strokes are generally much shorter than this and are proportional to the area being treated. For example, the length of the eyebrow can be divided into three different stroking areas.

DIRECTION

The general rule in any normal scraping action is to stroke downwards or outwards and to follow along the muscle fibres (not across them), but there are variations on this, depending on the body part.

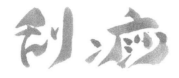

7

IS IT THE SAME FOR EVERYONE?

Too often people are left out of the equation in modern medicine. Modern drugs are designed for diseases not for people, and effectively ignore the infinite variations that exist among us. You take a pill for a headache; you do not take a pill for a person with a headache. There may be different reasons for that headache, and your reaction to the medicine may be different, but you are essentially seen in terms of the headache. Oriental medicine usually takes a more holistic view. That means that Gua sha is not used as a one-size-fits-all pill but is adapted to your needs as a person. With this is mind, there are two key ways to apply Gua sha on yourself.

STYLES OF TREATMENT
PURGING

If you have a cough or cold, your intention is essentially one of removal. Maybe you want to remove the tension in the trapezius muscle at your shoulder. Maybe you want to remove the mucous collecting in your lungs. Maybe you want to remove inflammation of your respiratory tract. In Oriental medicine terms, you want to remove the wind or cold or heat that has invaded your chest.

This is probably the most common use of Gua sha and often involves those tell-tale red marks on the skin. It consists of heavy pressure and rapid strokes in order to bring out as much *sha* as possible. We can refer to this as a purging technique, as your intention is the removal of stagnation and tension in the connective tissue.

You are metaphorically scraping the carrot skin from the carrot. Remember that this is about your intention of treatment and not about actually physically removing substances from the body. Removing heat from the body, when treating a fever, or removing wind, when treating the symptoms of a common cold, does not mean that it will materialize out of the skin in front of you like the genie in Aladdin's lamp. The process of removal is indicated by the petechiae marks on the skin, and the body will adjust its internal balance appropriately.

TONIFYING

There are times when *sha* does not come to the surface, even though you thought it would. Perhaps you are doing Gua sha over sore shoulders, but try as you may no petechiae appears. This does not mean that the treatment has no therapeutic value. Far from it. The tension that existed in the musculature and the connective tissue has still been released, and there very probably will be an improvement in the condition.

Gua sha is a proactive technique that has an effect not only on the movement of blood and *qi* and how the channels distribute them around the body but on the creation of new blood. This is how you might do Gua sha on your shoulders through your clothing at the end of a stressful day, for example, and even though no *sha* was involved with the *Gua*, it still improved the circulation through the shoulders and relieved the tension.

This is part of another use of the Gua sha, whereby you are not intending to bring sha to the surface of the skin. This involves an equally firm yet gentler technique. If you use Gua sha on your head for example, the strokes over the head have a very valuable therapeutic effect without any marking of the skin.

This gentler technique is known as a tonifying technique and consists of slow, moderate strokes which do not have to mark the skin to be effective. It has more of a strengthening and supporting action and has far greater relevance to certain areas of the body like the head and face.

A simple example of a tonifying technique is on coldness in the feet and hands. Usually this means a lack of circulation of blood and *qi* in the body, which has its origins somewhere in the balance of the organs. Your body may be energetically weak, in that there is just not the power to send enough energized blood all the way to the extremities on a constant basis. Or perhaps your body suffers from stagnation and obstruction, and the flow of blood is being slowed or blocked by problems elsewhere.

Whichever the case, the local circulation of blood and *qi* can be helped with Gua sha. Not the purging type but gentle strokes between the toes/fingers, over the top of the foot/hand and on the soles/palms of the feet/hands. The idea being an increase in local circulation will increase the feeling of warmth. Of course, there is more to improving poor circulation that this, but it will help to strengthen and support the body.

ADAPTING TREATMENTS

Bearing in mind the distinction between tonifying and purging in the use of Gua sha, it is very important to keep in mind the following guidelines when performing this technique:

PRESSURE

Start with light pressure as you stroke and increase it according to how comfortable it feels and what your intention is (purging or tonifying).

The amount of pressure used has a major impact on how the body

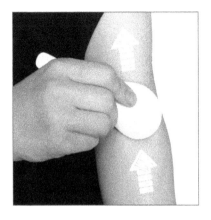

Image 28. Tonification technique

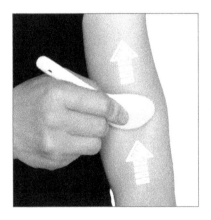

Image 29. Purging technique

reacts. Essentially, the more pressure you use, the more draining it is. Sometimes, this is a good thing in order to promote circulation or remove tension from the body, but if you feel generally weak, strong pressure should be avoided or you may feel weaker.

Light pressure is more associated with a strengthening and nourishing effect, but please note that it can still bring *sha* to the surface of the skin in some people.

SPEED

The same logic can be applied to the speed of the stroking action. A faster action is used to move or expel and a slower one to reinforce and strengthen. A faster stroke is therefore more purging and a slower stroke more tonifying.

ANGLE

The angle of the tool has an effect on the strength of treatment. The lower the angle facing the direction of the stroke, the stronger and more purging the Gua sha action is (image 28 and 29).

DURATION

The longer you stroke, the more internal movement you generate. So, again, if you are weak and exhausted, the length of time you stroke should be short.

In general, if your intention is to bring *sha* to the surface, about a dozen strokes in the same area should be enough for it to appear, although this varies with people. The longer you stroke, the more likely *sha* will appear. If it does appear, it is important to continue in the area around it, to ensure that all of the *sha* comes out. When no new spots appear on the skin in the area around it, then it is time to move on to another area.

For any kind of treatment, apply Gua sha for no more than 20 to 30 minutes.

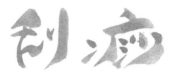

8

IS IT SAFE?

CONDITIONS

As mentioned in the WHO IS IT FOR? section, you need to be cautious about certain areas of the body and there are certain conditions which mean you should not use Gua sha techniques.

FEATURES

Any raised skin features like moles and spots should be covered with a finger of your other hand. Do not directly scrape over these features.

TOOLS

Although Gua sha has been practised for a long time, only very recently have concerns been raised about cross-contamination of Gua sha tools.[21] There remains, however, the potential for cross-contamination with a blood-borne virus such as Hepatitis B, Hepatitis C, or HIV if using the same tool on other people as is commonly done in clinical situations. This is because although there is no bleeding involved, it is thought that the scraping action involves the removal of skin matter containing blood cells.

For much of the contents of this book, this should not be an issue. Scraping through clothing for example does not involve direct contact with the skin; contact is minimal with light strengthening techniques that do not bring out *sha*; and treating yourself in the shower or bath is not that dissimilar to scrubbing with a sponge. There are many situations that I include in this book which make any risk negligible.

To be on the safe side however the obvious solution to avoid any issue of contamination is to minimize the risk of this by not sharing the tool with anyone else. If you are using the tool on yourself for self-treatment, cross-contamination may still potentially occur if you are not mindful about which surfaces you and the tool touch during and after the treatment. This is especially true if you use lubrication. It is best to have everything you need ready in front of you rather than touching and potentially contaminating things around you.

Cleaning

If the tool has scraped directly on the skin, then it needs to be cleaned after each treatment. In theory, the ideal way to clean a Gua sha tool to prevent cross-contamination is to sterilize the tool in an autoclave, the machine commonly found in dentists to sterilize the dental equipment. Other sterilization options include chemical sterilisation using a medical disinfectant such as PeraSafe, which being a sporicidal, tuberculocidal, virucidal, bactericidal, and fungicidal, will kill off just about anything. Which of course is part solution and part problem purely because it does kill everything, including the environment. The trouble with both of these methods, apart from the practicality of them, is that most tools used in Gua sha are made from materials that are not suitable for sterilization in an autoclave or with chemicals, like bone or horn.

A simple, practical cleaning solution to all this is to immerse your Gua sha tool in a solution of 1 part bleach and 9 parts water, or 7 parts alcohol and 3 parts water, for 10 minutes. Be careful not to leave the tool any longer because some materials, such as horn, bend when over-exposed to water or remain wet.

PART 3

HOW DO YOU USE GUA SHA ON YOUR BODY?

In this section the body has been divided into areas of treatment with Gua sha. When you stroke the surface of the skin, it is important to know what lies beneath, both in terms of muscles, tendons, and body tissues but also in terms of the channels and points of Oriental medicine. In this way you can explore how parts of the body are connected and the possible conditions to treat can make more sense.

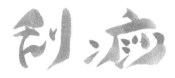

9

THE UPPER BODY

HEAD AREA

UNDER THE SKIN
Bones

The hard bone that protects the head is known as the cranium. Gua sha technique in this area is dominated by the fact that it lies so close to the skin. Strong pressure is therefore contraindicated.

Muscles & Tissues

When thinking of the head, you do not immediately think of muscles. There barely seems room for them, with the skull taking up most of the space in the head area. Thin muscle layers lie between the skin and connective tissue and the cranium bone. The most important, in terms of Gua sha, are the following:

△ The occipitalis muscle is at the back of the skull, above the lower edge of the occiput. It helps you move your scalp, raise your eyebrows, or wrinkle your forehead. These movements

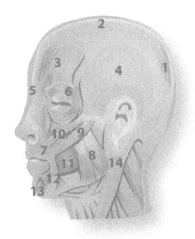

1. Occipitalis muscle
2. Galea aponeurotica tendon/fascia
3. Frontalis muscle
4. Temporalis muscle
5. Procerus muscle
6. Orbicularis oculi muscle
7. Orbicularis oris muscle
8. Masseter muscle
9. Zygomaticus muscles (zygomaticus minor and major)
10. Levator labii superioris muscle
11. Risorius muscle
12. Depressor muscles
13. Mentalis muscle
14. Sternocleidomastoid muscle

Image 30. Muscles and tissues of the head

are often connected to emotions, and there can be a surprising amount of tension stored here.

△ A broad, flat sheet of dense, fibrous connective tissue resembling a flat tendon, which stretches all the way over the top of the head, is known as the galea aponeurotica. Much like a helmet, it connects the occipitalis muscle at the back with the frontalis muscle at the forehead. Together these muscles are known as the epicranius muscle, and there are invariably sore areas dotted around it that become evident upon palpation.

△ The side of the head is covered by a different muscle known as the temporalis, which helps you open and close your jaw. This stretches from the temple area (hence the name) to behind the level of the ear. It too can store more tension than you might think.

Channels

The head area is crisscrossed by several channels, many of which begin at the face, flow over the head, then descend the trunk of the body.

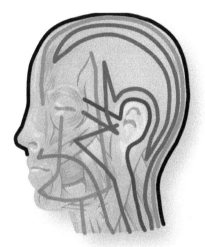

Image 31. Channels of the head

△ The centre line from the back of the head to just below the nose is called the Du or Governing channel (black). As it comes all the way up the spine and goes over the vertex of the head, it has a strong connection with problems associated with the head, such as dizziness and mental or emotional issues.

△ Parallel to this is the Bladder channel (dark blue), which starts to the side of the eye and flows back over the head all the way down to the little toe. It is the longest channel in the body, with a total of 67 points, and has a variety of functions. The nine head points on the Bladder channel are closely connected to the eyes and nose but also to psycho-emotional disorders.

△ The Gall bladder channel (dark green) zigzags its way over the side of the head and, like the Bladder channel, stretches right down to the feet. Due to its location on the head, it is often implicated in ear problems and headaches, especially those that affect the temples or around the eyes.

△ A branch of the Stomach channel (orange) also juts out into the corner of the head and features a point at the end that is often sore to touch and hugely beneficial for helping you concentrate and clear your head.

COMMON AILMENTS CONNECTED TO THIS AREA

Headaches, migraines, high blood pressure, dizziness, stress, depression, anxiety, nasal and facial disorders, ear and eye problems.

HEAD SEQUENCE

The following is a sequence of Gua sha scraping which, when done together, can have a very relaxing effect on the head (and also neck areas).

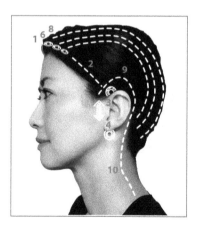

Image 32. Head sequence

1. Use a vibrate technique, but with the side of the tool, as the corner can be too harsh on the head area. Continue for about 10 seconds at each of the three points at the frontal hairline: one on the midline, one at the corner of the head, and one in between. Then repeat on the other side (image 32 and 33).

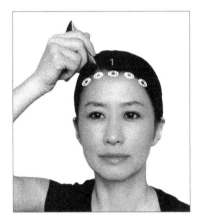

Image 33. Head sequence

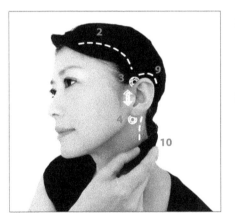

Image 34. Head sequence

2. Narrow stroke from the mid-point along and down to the top of the ear (image 34).
3. Place the side of the tool on the top attachment of the ear and narrow stroke on the head while pushing down the top of the ear. Move the tool forwards slightly, and narrow stroke the front of the ear (image 34).
4. Repeat this at the bottom attachment of the ear, this time pushing the bottom of the ear up. Follow it again with a narrow stroke at the front of the ear (image 34).

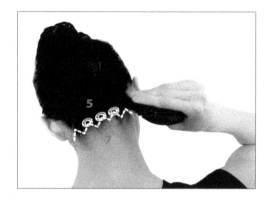

Image 35. Head sequence

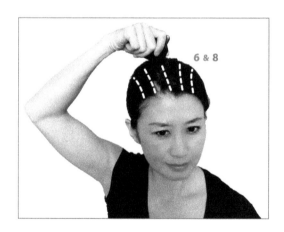

Image 36. Head sequence

5. Press the midpoint in the occiput at the back of the head. Then stroke one point either side, about three finger widths away in the muscle (image 35).
6. Wide stroke straight backwards towards the top of the head from each of the frontal points in 1 (image 36).
7. Stroke firmly and with short up and down movements along the length of the occiput using a vibrate technique.
8. As if combing your hair, use the tool to stroke back to the occiput from the points in 1, using short pressured wide strokes (image 36).
9. Wide stroke from the front of the ear around to the back of the ear. Use short firm strokes (image 32 & 34).
10. From the back of the ear continue the movement down the side of the neck (image 32 & 34).

Gua Sha

Face area

General caution

Be wary of Gua sha to the face—marks are not usually desirable, so lighter pressure and a more tonifying technique are preferable.

Under the skin
Bones

Certain bones in the face serve as guidelines to Gua sha. These include:

△   The orbital cavity, or eye socket, gives a natural smooth contour for stroking outwards: above, below, and around the socket.

△   Below the eye socket is the zygomatic bone, or cheek bone, the lower border of which provides another useful stroking line.

△   The mandible, or jaw bone, can give shape to strokes at the bottom of the face.

Muscles & tissues

Unlike muscles in other areas of the body, which attach to your bones, facial muscles are attached to other muscles or directly to your skin. This means that they are heavily influenced by your emotions and the faces that you pull naturally on a day-to-day basis.

The most relevant of these muscles for Gua sha are the following (see image 30 on page 78):

△   The forehead is dominated by the frontalis muscle and the temples by the temporalis, both of which are covered in the previous section. The frontalis is connected to the procerus muscle, which lies in the area between the eyebrows and the bridge of the nose and pulls the skin between the eyebrows downwards, allowing you to make the classic frowning expression of anger. Being stressed or unhappy can keep this muscle in a permanent state of tension.

△ The muscles that surround your eyes are known as the orbicularis oculi muscles. They allow the eyes to open and close and ensure they have enough moisture by compressing the tear duct.

△ There is also a similar-looking muscle surrounding the mouth called the orbicularis oris, which allows you to pucker your lips, as if to kiss. Both serve as a base for the attachments of smaller facial muscles.

△ The cheek is made up of the strong masseter muscle at the side, which controls the jaw and allows us to chew. This muscle often gets very tense. This is followed by a series of smaller muscles stretching from the mouth area to muscles in the temple, jaw, and eye. These muscles help you move your mouth, nose, and cheeks and help to form the nasolabial fold, the line from the nostrils to the outside of the mouth.

△ Two of these, the zygomaticus muscles, are parallel to each other but curiously have the opposite emotional effect. The zygomaticus major pulls the mouth up and out to make you appear happy and smiling, and the zygomaticus minor brings the lip backwards and outwards to make you look rather sad. Closer to the nose, the levator labii superioris muscles lift the upper lip and flare the nostril, giving you a slight snarl. Another is known as the risorius muscle, or laughing muscle, which pulls the mouth back to imitate a smile. As should be clear by now, these muscles are closely connected to the prevailing emotion that moves them.

△ The chin area is made up of the depressor muscles, which help you move down the corner of the mouth and bottom lip, and the mentalis muscle (known as the pouting muscle), which wrinkles your chin.

Channels & areas

Two important facets pertaining to the face must be considered in Oriental medicine. The first is that the face is considered to reflect the main organs and imbalances in the body, as can be seen in image 37.

The organs are reflected in areas in the face in descending order, with the Lungs at the forehead and, as you come down the nose, the Heart, then the Liver, with the Gall bladder on either side. At the tip of the nose are the two digestive organs, the Stomach and Spleen, and under them, the Bladder. In line with the eye, the Small intestines and Large intestines then lead on to the Kidneys at the side of the mouth.[22]

This means that changes in skin tone and skin features like lines, rashes, and marks can be more than just coincidence; they are perhaps telling you something important about what is happening in the balance of the organs in your body.

The second is that the face is crisscrossed with channels (see image 38) that lead down through the body to the feet - the Stomach channel, the Bladder channel, and the Gall bladder channel - and also some that head upwards and end at the face: the Ren and Du channels, the Small intestine channel, the Large intestine channel, and the Triple burner. Most of the points along these channels on the face have a local effect on the facial area: the ears, eyes, nose, and mouth.

△ The Stomach channel (orange) holds an important place in affecting the face and also problems inside the mouth, such as toothache, because it literally spans the whole face, from the eye to the chin to the corner of the jaw to the corner of the forehead. It is part of the *Yangming* cutaneous region which, along with the Large intestine channel (dark grey), dominates the facial region. This is why treatment on these channels farther away from the face can still have a direct local effect. In fact, Large intestine 4, or *Hegu*, is the single most important point to treat the face, and it is located in the muscle between the thumb and the index finger in the hand!

86

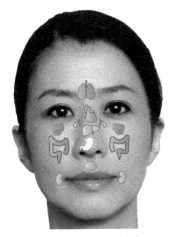

Image 37. Organs on the face

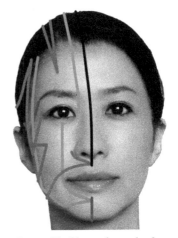

Image 38. Channels on the face

△ The other channels that run over the face have a variety of very important points. The Bladder channel (dark blue) begins with a point at the inside corner of the eye and goes up over the head. Only two points are actually located on the face, but both are very useful in supporting the eyes.

△ The Ren channel (light brown) ends at the chin, below the mouth, and the Du channel (black) actually ends in the top gum inside the mouth. Both contain potent points that affect the mouth and nose, but this is especially true of the final point of the Ren channel, as it is also the meeting point of the *Yangming* channels.

△ The Gall bladder channel (dark green) is mainly connected to the head, not to the face. However, with one point that stretches down to the mid forehead, one at the side of the ear, and the very first point on the channel just to the side of the eye, it can be just as important for the face. Along with the Small intestine channel (dark red) and the Triple burner channel (dark purple) which also pass by the attachment of the ear and close to the eye area, they are focused in the temple area and can be accessed easily with Gua sha.

Trigeminal neuralgia, sinus problems, earache, headache, migraines, depression, and eye disorders.

FACE SEQUENCE

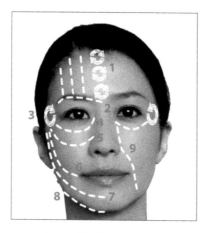

Image 39. Face sequence

1.   Place the corner of the instrument at the midpoint in between the eyebrows. Circle up the forehead to just below the natural hairline. Then repeat this line a second time. Move a finger width closer to the temple and repeat this circular movement up the forehead. Each line should go up parallel to the previous one until the edge of forehead. And each circular line should be repeated twice. It is very important that pressure it light and the movement is firm but gentle (image 39 and 40).

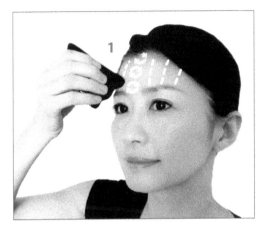

Image 40. Face sequence

2. Start in between the eyebrows and circle outwards along the
   eyebrow to end. Repeat again above the eyebrow and then
   below the eyebrow (image 41).

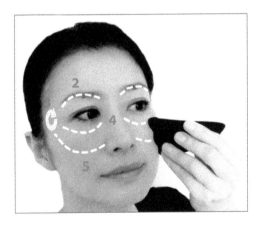

Image 41. Face sequence

3. Next move to the temple and press lightly with the corner of the tool while making a circular movement. Continue this for thirty seconds and repeat on both sides (image 41).

4. Start at the inside corner of eye and circle around the lower eye socket. Finish at the temple. Repeat on both sides (image 41).

5. Start at the side of the nose, around half way down and follow the cheek bone around to the temple. Repeat on both sides (image 41).

6. Start at corner of the lips and circle out and upwards to the temple. Repeat on both sides (image 42).

7. From the midpoint of the chin, circle outwards and upwards to the temple. Repeat on both sides (image 42).

8. Return to the midpoint of the chin but go lower, just below the jaw bone and follow it around until below the ear (image 42).

9. Circle from below the nasolabial groove to the sides of the nostrils. Circle upwards and at the bridge of the nose, follow the eye socket around again and finish at temples (image 39).

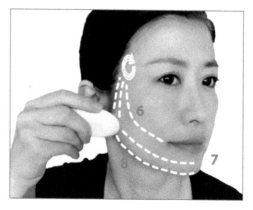

Image 42. Face sequence

The upper body

Neck and shoulder area

General caution

Avoid scraping directly at the front of the neck. The front does not have the muscular protection that the back and sides have, and the laryngeal prominence (otherwise known as the Adam's apple) is particularly vulnerable to damage.

Under the skin
Bones

Neck

Scraping down the back of your neck begins at the lower edge of the occipital bone which forms the back of the skull. The structure of the neck is then created by the cervical vertebrae (numbered from C1 to C7). When you turn your head from side to side the last vertebra of the neck (C7) moves while the next one down (T1) does not because it is attached to the first rib (see image 44 on page 94).

Caution

Be cautious when scraping down the cervical vertebrae, especially if you have pins and needles down your arm. This could mean a problem with the vertebrae and scraping should be avoided.

Shoulder (back)

The acromion process is the bony prominence at the top part of the shoulder blade towards the shoulder joint. It provides attachments for the deltoid and trapezius muscles and protrudes outwards meaning that you should be cautious of this when scraping the shoulder area.

From here slanting downwards towards the spine runs another protuberance called the spine of scapula. Above it is the trapezius muscle and below it, the deltoid. Be aware of its position and be cautious not to perform Gua sha directly on this bone. It hurts!

Shoulder (front)

The thin horizontal clavicle bones at the top of the chest attach to the acromion at the shoulder. Be mindful of scraping on the muscular areas and not directly on this bony area. Again the result may very well be pain!

Muscles & tissues

There are many small muscles in this heavily worked area but in terms of Gua sha the main ones are:

△ The sternocleidomastoid muscles, which help you rotate and move your head from side to side, sit obliquely down the sides of the neck. There is often tension here when there is neck stiffness or pain. Turn your head to the side and the muscle on the other side is easier to get to.

△ The splenius capitus muscles lie deeper at the back of the neck but can be directly accessed between the sternocleido-mastoid muscles and the trapezius muscles. This muscle can easily become tense or damaged as it helps to rotate and keep the head upright.

△ The levator scapula muscle lies at the side and back of the neck. It connects the neck and shoulder and is used to lift the shoulders and turn the head. It often heavily features in limited neck rotation.

△ The trapezius muscles, the upper part of which helps you lift your shoulder and support it when carrying something heavy, connect the back of the neck, the shoulders and the thorax. For this reason it can be very tense and sensitive to pressure.

△ The deltoid muscle gives the rounded shape at the top of the arm. It covers the shoulder joint and part of the scapula at the

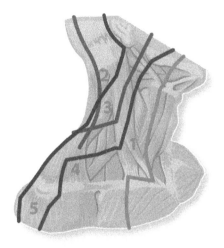

1. Sternocleidomastoid muscle
2. Splenius capitus muscle
3. Levator scapula muscle
4. Trapezius muscle
5. Deltoid muscle
6. Spine of scapula
7. Acromion process

Image 43. Muscles, tissues & channels in the neck (side)

back and helps to lift and rotate the arm. Prod around and it is not usually very difficult to find sore points in this muscle.

Channels

Apart from local pain in the neck and shoulder, scraping over this area can have a strong knock on effect on the head and body area. This is because the area is an important crossroads of channels coming up and down the trunk of the body and those heading up and down the arm. So many diverging channels means that, rather like the accumulation of leaves on the train track, it is an area that is prone to obstruction. It also means that treatment here to remove the blockage can have a strong effect both physically and emotionally by promoting greater circulation.

△ The Small intestine channel (dark red) cuts through the deltoid muscles and then the sternocleidomastoid muscles on its way up to the ear. Despite its name, it is not indicated for any digestive or intestinal problems but is instead an important

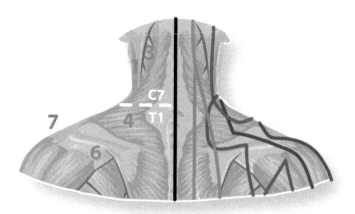

Image 44. Muscles, tissues & channels in the neck (back)

channel in any neck and shoulder disorder. Like the Large intestine channel which passes right through the heads of the deltoid muscle at the top of the arm and over the top of the trapezius muscle and the Triple burner channel which comes up the back of the arm through the triceps, over the acromion and over the top of the trapezius, some of the most potent points to treat are located not in the shoulder but lower down in the forearm and hand.

△ The Gall bladder channel (dark green) comes down the back of the neck to the height of the trapezius. This channel is particularly affected by stress and tends to contract the muscles around it. It is particularly responsive to Gua sha, not just locally in the trapezius and neck muscles but along the channel in the lower legs.

△ The Du channel (black) runs up the midline of the back of the body and so is closely connected to the spine. Key local points in the neck are actually in the gaps between the spinal vertebrae so treatment along the Du channel, while hugely beneficial, needs caution.

The upper body

Common ailments connected to this area

Neck/shoulder pain, dizziness, headaches, migraines, muscle tension, depression, anxiety and insomnia.

Neck & shoulder sequence

Be mindful that this is an area that gets very tense and can easily develop red marks on the skin during scraping. With any neck and shoulder treatment, begin at the top and work your way down.

1. Wide stroke down the side of the neck from below the ear along the sternocleidomastoid and other muscles (image 45).
2. Wide stroke across the top of the trapezius muscle towards the arm. Remember to be cautious with the acromion, the bony part at the end (image 45).

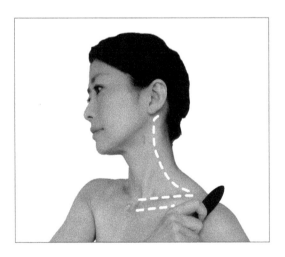

Image 45. Neck and shoulder sequence

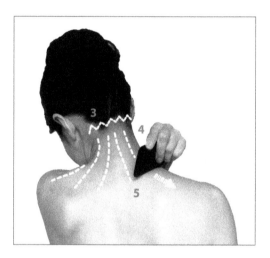

Image 46. Neck and shoulder sequence

3. Vibrate up and down along the full length of the lower edge of the occiput (image 46).
4. Wide stroke down the back of the neck in regular intervals. Gua sha practice in China has divided the neck into distinct scraping areas made up of six areas on either side from the midline below the occiput to the mastoid process, the corner of the jaw bone. You do not need to be as precise as this but cover the same area and it is important that your strokes are short, smooth and downwards (image 46).
5. Wide stroke into the trapezius muscle at the top part of the back (image 46).

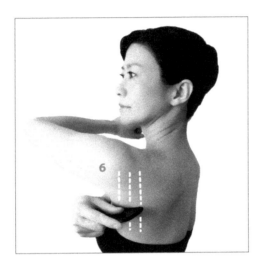

Image 47. Neck and shoulder sequence

6. Lift up your arm and rest it on your opposite shoulder. Wide stroke down the side of the trapezius muscle. This is an area that is often neglected when doing Gua sha connected with the shoulders but often brings out *sha* (image 47).

Gua Sha

Upper back area

For the purposes of convenience I have separated the back into two parts: the upper and the mid and lower. The idea being that with the latter it is possible to treat yourself. For treatment of the upper however, the practicalities are much more difficult and you probably need another pair of hands to help you.

Under the skin
Bones

- △ The spine in this area is made up of the thoracic vertebrae which can protrude in some people, so avoid scraping directly over the spine unless the vertebrae are sufficiently padded by soft tissue. Having said that, a common site of reaction on the skin is in the gaps between the vertebrae. These are the dips between the many bony protuberances known as the spinous processes.
- △ The scapula, otherwise known as the shoulder blade, is well padded by muscle but it can still be very sensitive to pressure, especially around the midpoint of the flat area.
- △ In particular be cautious with the scapular spine which is a ridge of bone, mentioned in the shoulder section, which runs along the top part of the scapula angled towards the spine. Scraping over this can be uncomfortable.
- △ The muscles have sufficient depth in the back so that scraping can be in a downwards direction over the rib area. Should you be very thin and there is little muscle or other soft tissue protecting your ribs, be cautious and follow the rib spaces across instead.

Muscles & tissues

△ The upper back is dominated by the trapezius muscle and much of the downward scraping between the spine and the scapula is over this muscle. It has already been mentioned in the shoulder and neck section and is a very common area for muscle soreness and tension.

△ The deltoid muscle connects the back to the top of the arm and with the rotator cuff muscles that cover the scapula area. The rotator cuff muscles help us move and stabilize the shoulder. This is another common area of accumulated tension.

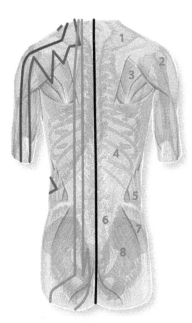

1. Trapezius muscle
2. Deltoid muscle
3. Rotator cuff muscles
4. Latissimus dorsi muscle
5. Abdominal oblique muscles
6. Thoracolumbar fascia
7. Gluteus medius muscle
8. Gluteus maximus muscle

Image 48. Muscles, tissues and channels on the back

CHANNELS

Three channels flow over and therefore influence the upper back.

△ The mid-line channel that runs up the spine is known as the Du or Governing channel (black) and contains important points close to the neck area for regulating heat and calming fever.

△ The Small intestine channel (dark red) which zigzags over the scapula on its way up to the neck, is primarily used for cooling heat and alleviating pain in the neck, shoulder and arm.

△ The Bladder channel (dark blue) which heads down the whole back is very much like the Small intestine channel in that it does not have much to do with the actual functioning of the bladder. It covers the *Taiyang* cutaneous region and is the most superficial of all the 'yang' channels. This means that when the body has to defend itself from environmental factors such as wind, heat and cold, it is the first to be affected. The points on the Bladder channel on the upper part of the back are very much focused on expelling these factors and regulating the lungs. Near the bottom of the scapula they are more focused on regulating the heart and 'spirit'.

COMMON AILMENTS CONNECTED TO THIS AREA

Colds, flu, coughs, asthma, bronchitis, depression, anxiety, sinus problems, eye problems, neck and shoulder pain and tight chest.

UPPER BACK SEQUENCE

Gua sha practice in China divides the upper back into crisscross scraping areas known as *Jianjiahuan*. Five lines run down the back - one on the midline, one half way between the midline and the edge of the scapula, and one in-between these two on both sides. As far as channels and points go, these correspond to the Du channel on the midline, a line of points known as the *Huatuojiaji* points close to the spine and the inner Bladder channel.

THE UPPER BODY

NOTE: The upper back area is very difficult to treat on yourself. I have included it here in case you wish to use this information to get some help. This book is designed for treating yourself and if you are treating someone else please note the following:

- The petechiae marks on the skin that are sometimes present after Gua sha can be misunderstood and interpreted wrongly by some people.
- Ideally you should have some kind of hands-on training as there is a difference between doing it on yourself and on another person.
- The issue of cross-contamination of tools and surfaces as featured in 'Is IT SAFE?' on page 71.

This downward movement is combined with an outwards sideways movement across the upper back. Eight zones are used and correspond to following the rib spaces from T1 to T9, midway down the back.

In practical terms, you do not need to follow this protocol too strictly. Generally scraping down the back next to the spine, down the two Bladder channels and outwards at the sides will produce good therapeutic results. The idea is not to achieve lines but areas of treatment. Remember that should *sha* come to the surface it is best to stroke around it, whether or not it fits in with any imagined linear sequence. Keep the strokes downwards and outwards.

1. Begin by lightly scraping down next to the spine. Remember that the strokes are short and repeated (See image 49).
2. Wide stroke down the mid area between the shoulder blades and the spine.
3. Wide stroke down the muscles close to the edge of the shoulder blades.
4. At the sides wide stroke outwards. Remember to go lightly over the scapula itself.

Repeat on both sides. This is especially true in cases of tightness and pain on one side of the body as there is often a corresponding obstruction on the other side.

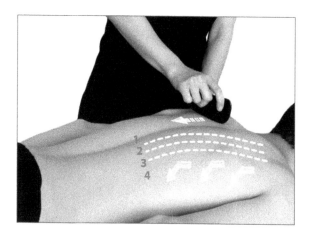

Image 49. Upper back sequence

The upper body

Chest area

Under the skin
Bones

△ The top of the chest is bordered by the clavicle which sits horizontally on either side of the midline. Be careful not to scrape directly on this but instead above and below it.

△ The sternum is the flat bone in the middle of the chest - although there is little in the way of softened protection it can still be scraped down.

△ Avoid scraping downwards over the ribs. Instead scrape following the rib spaces outwards from the centre.

△ At the bottom of the sternum there is a part that juts out called the xiphoid process. In some people it can be extended so avoid putting too much pressure on this area.

Muscles & tissues

△ The pectoralis major muscle, which moves the arm across the body, covers most of the upper chest from the sternum outwards. It is an area that frequently becomes tense and brings out *sha* on the skin.

△ At the sides of the chest from around the nipple level down lie the external abdominal obliques. These help to pull the chest downwards and are often connected to the feeling of tension and tightness in the chest.

△ Intercostal muscles are located between each rib and help expand and contract the thoracic cavity and so help in the

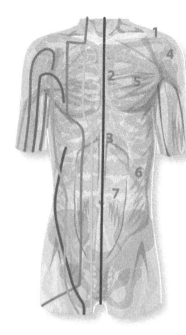

1. Clavicle bone
2. Sternum bone
3. Xiphoid process
4. Deltoid muscle
5. Pectoralis muscle
6. External abdominal oblique muscle
7. Rectus abdominus muscle

Image 50. Muscles, bones and channels on the front

action of breathing. Stroking between the ribs allows you to affect these muscles.

CHANNELS

△ The top corner of the chest, where the pectoralis major muscle meets the arm, is the Lung channel (light grey) and it is often tender especially when you have a cold, the flu or any respiratory condition.

△ The Ren channel (brown) runs up the centre line of the sternum and points along this channel are often a source of tenderness. Parallel to this, a short distance on either side, is the Kidney channel (light blue) and points in this area affect what is known as the 'spirit' in Oriental medicine and can help depression, anxiety and other problems connected to the head.

△ The middle area either side of the sternum is where the Stomach channel (orange) flows down the body. It follows an imaginary line running down from the middle of the clavicle through the nipple. Please note the caution for Gua sha at the beginning of this section (on page 103).

△ Further out at the sides of the body below the arm joint runs the end of the Spleen channel (yellow). This area is often neglected in Gua sha treatments but there is a surprising amount of tension stored here.

Common ailments connected to this area

Respiratory disorders, asthma, coughs, colds, flu, depression, anxiety, stress-related symptoms and reflux disorder.

GUA SHA

CHEST SEQUENCE

1. Start at the top of the sternum bone and wide stroke down. Stay on the bone and do not veer on to the ribs (image 51).
2. Narrow stroke outwards along the bottom of the clavicle. It is a sensitive area and any tender points can be lightly pressed (image 51).
3. Narrow stroke and follow the spaces between the ribs with outward strokes away from the centre line. If *sha* comes to the surface avoid only following the line but stroke the area around it. Return to the sternum each time you move down.

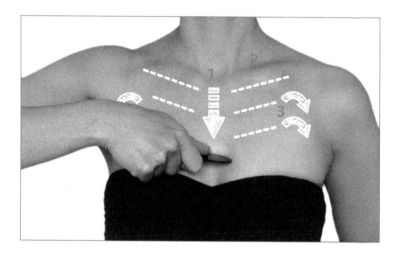

Image 51. Chest sequence

The upper body

Arms

Under the skin
Bones

Upper Arm
△ Avoid the bony parts in the elbow area - the olecranon (the tip of the elbow) at the back, the medial epicondyle of the humerus on the inside (the ulna nerve comes close to the bone here and it is often painfully referred to as the funny bone) and the lateral epicondyle of the humerus on the outside.

△ Stroke above and below the elbow joint, not actually on the bony joint itself. The inside part of the elbow joint is usually slapped with a Gua sha tool in China (ouch!) in order to encourage sha but this technique thankfully does not feature here.

Lower arm
△ The ulna (little finger side) and radius (thumb side) bones make up the lower arm. The edge of the ulna can be felt if you lift your lower arm vertically in front of you. Direct contact should be avoided when scraping.

△ Stop before the heads of the bones at the wrists, known as the styloid processes of the radius and ulna. There is little but bone and tendon here.

Muscles & tissues

Upper Arm
△ Scraping over the upper arm is relatively straightforward as the muscle mass usually provides a soft base all the way around the arm.

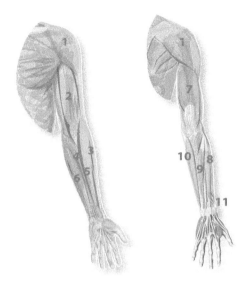

1. Deltoid muscle
2. Biceps muscle
3. Brachioradalis muscle
4. Palmarus longus muscle
5. Flexor carpi radialis muscle
6. Flexor carpi ulnaris muscle
7. Triceps muscle
8. Extensor digitorum muscle
9. Extensor carpi radialis longus muscle
10. Extensor and flexor carpi ulnaris muscle
11. Pollicis brevis and longus muscles

Image 52 & 53. Muscles and tissues on the arm

△ The top of the arm/shoulder bulks out with the deltoid muscle which comes down the arm in an inverted triangle. The deltoid muscle allows the arm to move in a rotational movement and is used when you walk and swing your arms. It is a muscle that can carry with it a lot of tension and features strongly in Gua sha treatment around this area.

△ The biceps, which help to bend the elbow and twist the forearm, then connect the top of the arm to the elbow joint at the front and the triceps, which work in the opposite direction, at the back. Both are of course well-used muscles which can benefit greatly from Gua sha.

Lower arm

Inside

△ The upper bulk below the elbow on the thumb side is the brachioradalis muscle. On the other side, the flexor carpi ulnaris muscle comes down the little finger side of the forearm and attaches to the wrist. The flexor carpi radialis and the palmaris longus cover the mid section and are the two prominent tendons that lead into the middle of the wrist joint. Move your hand up and down and you should see them clearly. Remember the closer you are to the wrist joint, the less muscle mass to cushion the stroking.

Outside
△ The outside of the forearm is a collection of long thin muscles leading into the hand. The largest of these is the extensor digitorum which runs down the middle of the back of the forearm and connects to, and moves, the fingers.
△ On the little finger side of this are the extensor and flexor carpi ulnaris muscles and on the thumb side, the bulk at the top is the brachioradialis followed by the extensor carpi radialis longus. These all affect the movement of the hand and wrist. Closer to the wrist joint, the short pollicis brevis and longus affect the thumb.

CHANNELS
Inside of the arm
△ The Lung channel (light grey) runs down the outside of the biceps muscle and down the radial side of the arms to the outside of the thumb. It affects local arm pain but has a strong influence over the respiratory system and especially colds, coughs and flu symptoms. It begins in the chest and therefore can also influence the chest muscles and feelings of stuffiness in the chest.
△ The Heart channel (light red) runs down the inside of the biceps and then down the flexor carpi ulnaris tendon to the wrist. It influences local pain in this part of the arm but also

anxiety and sleep problems.

△ The Pericardium channel (light purple) starts in the chest and heads down the inside arm through the centre of the biceps muscle. It then continues down the centre of the forearm to the wrist between the palmaris longus and the flexor carpi radialis. It has a strong effect on anxiety, the heart, the chest and on calming the stomach.

Outside of the arm

△ The Triple burner channel (dark purple) begins at the ring finger, goes over the back of the hand and up the arm between the ulna and radius bones, next to the extensor digitorium muscle. At the elbow it goes over the olecranon and then runs up the centre line of the triceps at the back of the arm to the shoulder. It influences local shoulder and arm pain and also

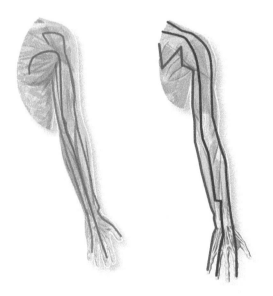

Image 54 & 55. Channels on the arm

ear pain.

△ The Small intestine channel (dark red) starts at the little finger and heads down the side of the arm, along the flexor carpi ulnaris muscle, through the gap between the olecranon and the medial epicondyle of the humerus and up inside the arm to the lower edge of the deltoid muscle where the arm attaches to the body. It influences local arm and elbow pain and also muscular shoulder problems and a sore neck.

△ The Large Intestine channel (dark grey) begins at the index finger and follows the extensor carpi radialis longus muscle along edge of the radius, over the elbow and the brachioradialis muscle and up through the outside of the biceps to the centre line of the deltoid muscle. It is important for local pain at the elbow and shoulder but as it also extends through the neck to the face it has considerable influence over a sore throat, toothache and headache.

COMMON AILMENTS CONNECTED TO THIS AREA

Shoulder, elbow and arm pain, heart conditions, lung and respiratory problems, sore throat, sore neck, chest tightness, toothache, headache and migraines.

ARM SEQUENCE

The general rule is to always scrape downwards or outwards but in fact strokes can go in either direction along the arms, depending on what position you are in and how you are treating. Strokes can follow the direction of channels or muscle fibres up and down but not across them in a sideways motion. Generally in a purging treatment scrape towards the hand. In tonifying treatments the movement is more upwards and supporting.

1. Wide stroke along the outside of the upper and lower arm. Do not stroke over the bony part of the elbow and stop before the wrist (image

56).

2. Wide stroke along the inside of the upper and lower arm. Also do not stroke over the bony part of the elbow and stop before the wrist (image 57).

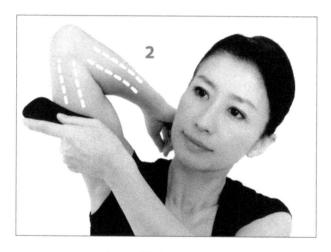

Image 56. Arm sequence

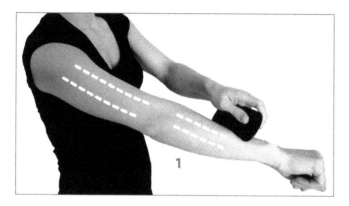

Image 57. Arm sequence

The upper body

Hands

Under the skin
Bones

The hands contain a total of 27 bones but it is the long, thin ones which are most relevant to Gua sha. These are the five metacarpals in the body of the hand and the phalanges in each of the fingers.

Muscles & tissues
Palm

The muscle bulk under the thumb is known as the thenar eminence. It is a collection of small muscles (the pollicis muscles) which allow the thumb its free movement.

On the other side are a collection of muscles which lead to and control the little finger. These are the digiti minimi muscles. The middle

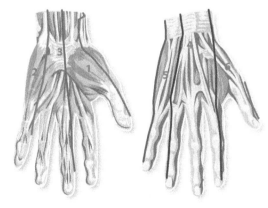

1. Thenar eminence
2. Digiti minimi muscles
3. Transverse carpal ligament
4. Extensor digitorum muscle
5. Extensor digiti minimi muscle
6. Extensor pollicis longus muscle

Image 58 & 59. Muscles, tissues & channels in the hand

part of the palm of the hand is a flat tendon which is a continuation of the palmaris longus muscle that goes into the arm, called the transverse carpal ligament. Gua sha treatment to the hand generally covers all these muscles.

Back of the hand

The back of the hand contains a group of extensor muscles and tendons which help it bend. The main ones stem from the elbow area and run all the way to the middle three fingers and little finger. These are called the extensor digitorum and extensor digiti minimi respectively. The thumb has its own shorter muscle, the extensor pollicis longus which helps it straighten out.

CHANNELS

The hand is also a busy area for channels. Three channels end and three channels start in the hand. This is important to know because the points at the extreme end of channels are often potent in terms of their effects on the rest of the body.

The three that start in the hand are the Small intestine (dark red), Large intestine (dark grey) and the Triple burner (dark purple) and all three contain points that have strong effects on problems associated with the other end of the channel. The Small intestine channel which goes up to the ear, has a strong influence over neck problems and key treatment points are located in the hand. Hand points along the Large intestine channel, which goes all the way up to the side of the nose, have a strong effect on the head and face. And hand points on the Triple burner channel, which ends near the eye, clear heat and fevers.

The three channels which end in the hand are the Heart (light red), Pericardium (light purple) and Lung (light grey) and they flow down the inside of the arm. All three come from the chest area and have powerful points to affect the chest, the heart, the respiratory system and the 'spirit' (psychological problems).

The upper body

Much of the body is reflected in the hand so it can affect a range of conditions but in particular a sore neck and shoulder, headache, migraine, anxiety, depression, insomnia, cold hands and feet, common cold, flu and fever.

Hand sequence
Palm
1. Narrow stroke with short strokes from the wrist along the thenar eminence below the thumb.
2. Narrow stroke in a similar fashion along the palm of the hand towards each of the fingers.
3. Narrow stroke along the side of the digiti minimi muscle below the little finger.
4. Narrow stroke with short pressured strokes along the sides of each fingers towards to finger tips.

Back of hand
5. Narrow stroke from the wrist between the metacarpal bones to the webs of the fingers. At each of the webs, press for five to ten seconds between the gap between the knuckle and the end of the web.

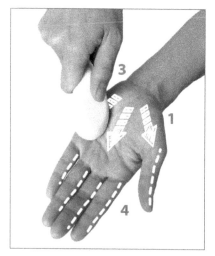

Image 60. Hand sequence

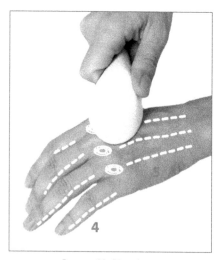

Image 61. Hand sequence

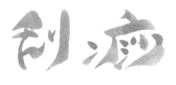

10

THE LOWER BODY

MID AND LOWER BACK AREA

This area is often affected when you have back ache, partly due to its importance in how we move and bend but also as it contains key points and areas connected with the major organs in the body. It is easy to presume that pain in your back is caused by a problem in the spine area or muscle strain, but the muscles in this area can also become tense as a reflection of an internal imbalance in these organs.

UNDER THE SKIN
Bones
△ This part of the back consists of a continuation of the thoracic vertebrae, the five lumbar vertebrae and the flat sacrum bone below. When you come to the sacrum, located above the area between the buttocks, there is less body tissue to cushion Gua sha so stroke accordingly.
△ The ribs in this area are called floating ribs because on one end they are attached to the spine but at the other there is no

attachment to the sternum like other ribs, instead they stretch out into the posterior abdominal muscles. You might come across the bottom rib towards the sides of the lower back and the area around it can be tender (more from the fact that the point Gall bladder 25 or *Capital gate* lies at the end of it than any issue with the rib).

Muscles & tissues

△ The triangular shape of the latissimus dorsi cuts across the mid back to the spine like a sail in the wind. It is attached to the spine by the thoracolumbar fascia which stretches all the way to the bottom of the sacrum. This muscle controls the shoulder joint and helps you to pull your arm back as you might do when doing the front crawl in a swimming pool. It is a very large and well-used muscle and because of this it is often very tight. It is usually fairly easy to find sore points (see image 48 on page 99).

△ Lower down at the beginning of the hip area the latissimus dorsi gives way to the external oblique abdominals which normally feature in the front of the body and help you to twist. This is the area that can be hidden by 'love handles'.

△ Below this are the powerful buttock muscles called the gluteus medius and the gluteus maximus. When scraping downwards in the lower back it is important for the final strokes to go into this muscle for the scraping action to be smooth and penetrating.

Channels

△ The mid and lower back continues to be dominated by the Bladder channel (dark blue) which flows down the central part of the back either side of the Du channel (black). The mid-back points on the Bladder channel are connected to the two digestive organs (the Stomach and Spleen) and also the

Liver and Gall bladder. The lower back points are then more used to treat lower back problems, Kidney issues and organs in the lower part of the body like the intestines and the uterus (see image 48 on page 99).

△ The sides of the mid and lower back are covered by the *Shaoyang* cutaneous region and influenced by the Gall bladder channel (dark green). This channel has a strong connection with *qi* circulation and muscle tension and also problems arising in the head area such as headaches, ear or eye problems.

COMMON AILMENTS CONNECTED TO THIS AREA

Local back pain, stomach or abdominal discomfort, bloating, constipation, diarrhoea, bloating, nausea, menstrual disorders, cystitis, intestinal disorders such as IBS or colitis, gallstones and leg, knee or foot pain.

MID & LOWER BACK SEQUENCE

1. Start at the mid-back and wide stroke down the centre of the back close to the spine, towards the sacral area (image 62). Keep each stroke normal length (between the length and width of your hand).
2. Wide stroke down an imaginary line taken from the midpoint of distance between the spine and the edge of the scapula. At the bottom stroke into the buttock muscles.
3. Wide stroke down an imaginary line taken from the edge of the scapula. At the bottom, stroke into the buttock muscles.
4. Wide stroke downwards and outwards at the sides.
5. At the sacrum stroke downwards and outwards. Be cautious with pressure if it is bony here.

Use press techniques on any tight, tender areas, especially when wide stroke techniques cause discomfort.

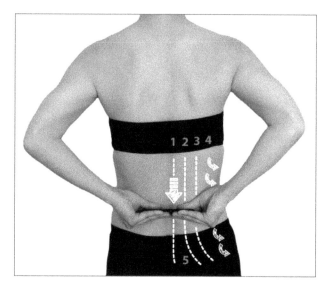

Image 62. Mid & Lower back sequence

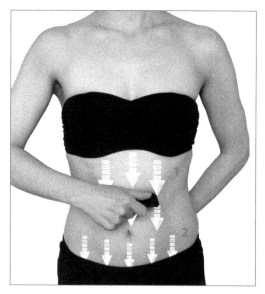

Image 63. Stomach & abdominal sequence

THE LOWER BODY

STOMACH & ABDOMINAL AREA

CAUTION
Be careful when practicing Gua sha on this part of the body. It does not have the bone infrastructure to support strong stroking. Also keep in mind never to do Gua sha on your abdomen if you are pregnant.

UNDER THE SKIN
Muscles & tissues

The obvious muscular place to start is the rectus abdominus muscle, otherwise known as the six-pack. This takes up much of the central area of the stomach and abdominal area and allows you to bend your back (see image 50 on page 104).

The other large muscles are the flat side muscles known as the external abdominal obliques and they help you twist and bend the spine.

CHANNELS
△ Scraping this area covers a neat row of channels. The center-line is the Ren channel (brown) which runs up the middle of the body towards the face. The points below the belly button are very much about the kidneys, bladder and uterus and above more concerned with digestion.

△ Close to this mid line on either side is the Kidney channel (light blue) which follows a similar pattern to the Ren channel above. And also like the Du points, most of the Kidney points in this area are connected with regulating the organs in this part of the body

△ Across to the edge of the rectus abdominus muscle is the Stomach channel (orange) which in this area has a strong influence on the intestines.

△ The Spleen channel (yellow) is further out to the side and travels up through the external abdominal oblique muscles.

This is an often overlooked but common site for accumulated muscular tension.

COMMON AILMENTS CONNECTED TO THIS AREA

Bloating, constipation, diarrhoea, menstrual pain and intestinal problems.

STOMACH & ABDOMINAL SEQUENCE

1. In China there is a set stroking directions for this area of the body known as *Sanwangua*. It consists of scraping down the midline of the body from the bottom of the sternum to the belly button. Then a line on both sides about three finger widths from the midline or half way from the midline to the outer edge of the abdomen muscles. These correspond to the Ren channel and the Stomach channels (image 63).

2. Also *Fubuwudaigua* which consists of an extension of the above but lower down the abdomen. Instead of three lines there are five with the extra line following the Spleen channel at the outer edge of the abdomen muscle (image 63).

While this is a useful sequence, in practical terms you can be flexible. It is important to respond to the shape of your body. Include also an outwards movement at the sides.

The lower body

Buttocks, hips & leg area

Under the skin
Bones

△ While most of the femur bone is hidden in the leg, the top protrudes outwards before it forms part of the hip joint. This boney part is known as the greater trochanter of the femur and you can feel it at the top of the sides of the leg. Excess pressure here can be sore.

△ The patella, or knee cap, has little to soften direct pressing so avoid using Gua sha directly on this bone.

△ There are two long bones in the lower leg. The thicker one on the big toe side is the tibia and next to this is the thin fibula. If you feel down the front of the lower leg, it is usually very easy to make out the edge of the tibia bone. Be aware that direct stroking on this bone can be painful.

△ Both bones become more prominent towards the ankle where the tibia curves out to form the medial malleolus on the inside and the fibula forms the lateral malleolus on the outside. This is where the ankle joint begins. There is very little soft tissue in this area so be cautious when stroking here.

Muscles & tissues
Upper leg: back

△ The buttocks and the side of the hip area are dominated by the gluteal group of muscles - the top by the gluteus medius, the back the gluteus maximus and the side the tensor fascia lata. There is often soreness at points at the side of these muscles.

△ Further down into the leg, the back group of muscles are called the hamstring muscles (the semitendinosus, semimembranosus and biceps femoris muscles), and they help to bend

123

(flex) the knee. They do this because they connect to the sides of the knee below the knee joint.

UPPER LEG: FRONT

△ The front and outside muscles of the thigh are grouped together as the quadriceps femoris muscles which help to bend (extend) the knee. You may not notice the build up of tension and soreness in these muscles but prod around and there are invariably tender areas especially towards the side of the thigh.

△ On the front and inside, a long, thin muscle crosses the thigh from the outside of the hip to below the inside of the knee. This is the sartorius muscle which helps you rotate your thigh, bend your knee and sit with your legs crossed.

LOWER LEG: BACK

△ Scraping the top half of the back of the leg is over the calf muscles - the gastrocnemius which help to bend the knee and to push the body forward when you walk and the soleus muscles which allows you to stand on the ball of your foot. This is a common sight of muscle cramping and tension.

△ Half way down the back of the leg this changes to the tendon of the gastrocnemius, a central band that leads down to the Achilles tendon. The soleus muscle becomes more prominent either side of this the further you head towards the ankle.

LOWER LEG: INSIDE

△ Below the knee, lie the attachments to important muscles that go up into the thigh such as the sartorius and the semitendinosus. This makes the area around the knee very important in terms of movement.

△ This is then followed by the sides of the large gastrocnemius or calf muscles. And then half way down the soleus which is squeezed between the tendon of the gastrocnemius and the tibia bone.

LOWER LEG: OUTSIDE

△ The tibialis anterior muscle, which allows you to bend and invert the foot, runs on the outside of the leg all the way from the knee to the bones in the foot. Beside this are long strips of muscle which stretch right down the leg - the extensor digitorum longus, the peroneus longus (higher) and brevis (lower).

CHANNELS

△ Three channels flow up the leg from the foot: the Liver (light green), the Spleen (orange) and the Kidney channel (light blue). They all follow the inside of the leg up through the soleus and gastrocnemius muscles to the knee and then through the inside thigh muscles to the groin area. All three meet at a point about four finger widths above the medical malleolus in the soleus muscle. This important point is called Spleen 6 or *Three yin meeting* and it is considered to have wide reaching effects in the body.

△ Three channels also flow down the leg which have travelled all the way through the body from the head. Two of these are commonly connected with hip and sciatic leg pain: The Bladder channel (dark blue) which runs down the centre-line of the back of the leg, and the Gall bladder channel (dark green) which runs all the way down the outside of the leg.

△ The other channel is the Stomach channel (yellow) which comes down the thigh, passes over the outside of the knee and through the tibius anterior muscle to the middle of the ankle. This channel actually has a point in the knee joint so is often indicated with knee problems.

1. Gluteus maximus
2. Gluteus medius
3. Sacrum
4. Greater trochanter of the femur
5. Semitendinosus (hamstring) muscle
6. Biceps femoris (hamstring) muscle
7. Semimembranosus (hamstring) muscle
8. Gastrocnemius muscle
9. Soleus muscle
10. Achilles tendon
11. Quadriceps femoris muscles
12. Sartorius muscle
13. Gastrocnemius muscle
14. Soleus muscle
15. Tibialis anterior muscle
16. Extensor digitorum longus muscle
17. Peroneus longus and brevis muscles

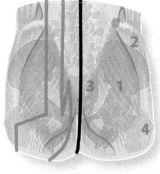

*Image 64. Muscles, tissues &
channels of the buttocks*

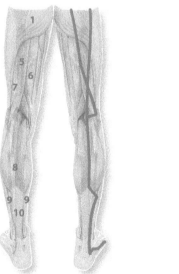

*Image 65. Muscles, tissues &
channels of the legs (back)*

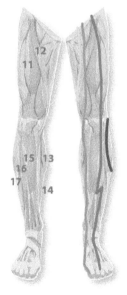

*Image 66. Muscles, tissues &
channels of the legs (front)*

The lower body

Lower back pain, hip pain, menstrual disorders, bladder disorders, sciatic pain, intestinal problems, prostate and genital problems, leg and knee weakness or pain, leg cramps, sciatic pain, stomach discomfort, headaches and ear or hearing problems.

BUTTOCKS, HIP AND LEG SEQUENCE

1. Wide stroke across the buttocks from the sacrum downwards and outwards into the upper leg (image 67).
2. Wide stroke down the side of hip area. Be cautious with the head of the femur bone which can stick out at the top of the leg (image 67).
3. Wide stroke down the inside of the upper and lower leg. Avoid the bony knee area (image 68).
4. Wide stroke down the outside and back of the upper and lower leg. Avoid the bony knee area (image 69).

Use a press technique on any tender points.

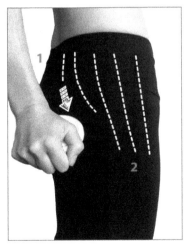

Image 67. Buttocks, hips & legs sequence

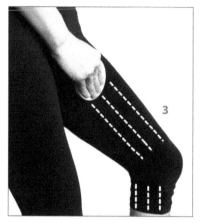

*Image 68. Buttocks, hips
& legs sequence*

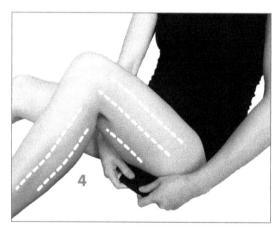

*Image 69. Buttocks, hips
& legs sequence*

The lower body

Feet area

Under the skin
Bones

The foot contains a total of 26 bones, the largest of which is the calcanium at the heel of the foot. This bone provides the attachments for many of the muscles that help you move your feet.

The main body of the foot is made up of five long metatarsal bones which lead onto the phalanges bones in the toes. For Gua sha these are more an issue on the top of the foot rather than the sole and you should take care not to scrape directly on bone.

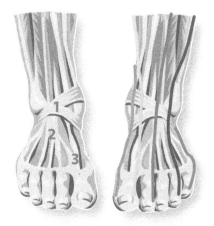

1. Inferior extensor retinaculum sheath
2. Extensor digitorum tendons
3. Extensor hallusis longus tendon

Image 70. Muscles, tissues & channels of the feet

Muscles & tissues

- △ The thick Achilles tendon stretches from the calf muscles down to the calcanium at the back of the foot. Gua sha in this area should be with light pressure.
- △ The sole of the foot is covered by the dense fibrous tissue

known as plantar aponeurosis which provides a comfortable cushion for Gua sha.

△ The instep (the big toe side) contains the thick abductor hallusis muscles which help to move the big toe and along the outstep (the little toe side) the abductor digiti minimi controls the movement of the little toe.

△ The top of the foot contains extensor digitorum tendons which connect the extensor digitorum muscle of the leg with the toes. The big toe has a separate tendon called the extensor hallusis longus tendon. These tendons are neatly tied into place by two sheaths of connective tissue that cross over the ankle, the inferior and superior extensor retinaculum. Pressure should be light in this area.

CHANNELS

△ The Kidney channel (light blue) is the only channel to start on the sole of the foot. Although being at the far extremity of the body, this point is actually used to treat conditions normally associated with the other end of the body such as dizziness, sore throat, insomnia and high blood pressure.

△ The soles of the feet are seen as a microsystem in Oriental medicine and using Gua sha on the soles of the feet can have additional effects on the body.

△ The rest of the Kidney channel goes through the abductor hallusis muscle at the instep and then circles the medial malleolus at the ankle. The points along here are generally strengthening for your core energy levels.

△ Two other channels start at the foot and head up to the chest area. Both the Spleen (yellow) and the Liver (light green) channels start at the nail bed of the big toe. The Spleen channel begins on the inside of the nail bed and follows the instep before heading up in front of the medial malleolus and the Liver channel starts on the other side of the big toe, goes up between the first and second metatarsal bones and then closely follows the Spleen channel over the ankle. This area contains potent points for treating conditions higher up in the body such as headache, anxiety and digestive problems.

△ Three channels finish in the feet. The Stomach channel (yellow) actually starts at the eye and travels all the way down the body over the midpoint of the ankle joint and then down through the middle of the foot to the start of the nail bed of the second toe. The Gall bladder channel (dark green) travels in front of the lateral malleolus and down the side of the foot to the nail bed of the fourth toe. And the Bladder channel (dark blue) comes down the edge of the Achilles tendon, under the lateral malleolus and along the side of the foot to the nail bed of the little toe.

△ All three of these channels have an effect on the areas in the body that each of them passes through on their way to the foot. For example, the Bladder channel in this area is heavily connected to back pain, the Stomach channel to stomach heat and the Gall bladder channel to clearing tension and stagnation.

COMMON AILMENTS CONNECTED TO THIS AREA

Plantar fasciitis, local foot pain, leg and foot swelling or puffiness, cold hands and feet, headaches, insomnia, high blood pressure and anxiety.

FOOT SEQUENCE

Sole of the foot

1. Wide stroke along the length of the sole starting from the heel area. Stop before the toes and repeat several times so that you cover the width of the sole (image 71).

2. Press the Kidney point for five to ten seconds. It is about a third of the distance between the bottom of the second toe

and the heel.

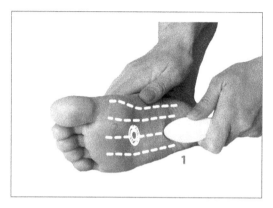

Image 71. Foot sequence

Sides of the foot

3. Narrow stroke along the instep (the abductor hallusis muscle) towards the ankle (image 72).
4. Narrow stroke along the outstep (the abductor digiti minimi muscle) towards the ankle (image 73).
5. Narrow stroke around the bottom of the ankle on both sides of the leg (image 72).

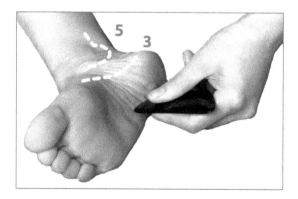

Image 72. Foot sequence

Top of the foot

6. Narrow stroke or circle at equal spacing down the foot from the ankle to the four webs between the toes. Press into the gap between the toes for five to ten seconds before moving on to the next (image 73).

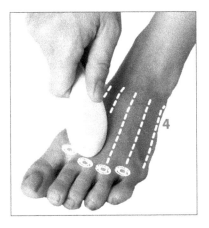

Image 73. Foot sequence

PART 4

HOW CAN YOU HELP YOUR HEALTH?

This section details some of the more common treatments using Gua sha based on my own clinical practice and on Chinese and Japanese ideas of treatment. They are not designed to be definitive and as we are all individuals may need adjustment for the treatment to fit the person. At the very least they should give you a useful starting point.

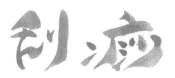

11

USE GUA SHA TO STAY HEALTHY

You may be coughing, spluttering, hobbling or limping around but an important point to keep in mind is that you do not need to be suffering aches and pains or the symptoms of a cold to use Gua sha techniques.

Good health is not just the absence of symptoms. Oriental medicine sees ill health as an imbalance and although symptoms tell us about imbalances, you do not have to have symptoms to be imbalanced. The idea is to find these imbalances before they become full on symptoms of an illness.

In my craftsman days in Japan I would often wander the primeval forests of my island home and stand in awe of the ancient trees. These were not any old trees but many thousands of years old and they had a presence far beyond being a tree. When Tolkien wrote about the 'Ents' in the Lord of the Rings he was thinking about trees like this. Some of them were wrinkled like a tired old face and others so weather beaten that the bark looked like elephant skin. Most of them looked a picture of health with blooming flowers and fresh green leaves and if you whisked past en route to the top of the mountain range, you would not be any the wiser.

The thing is that some of them were actually dead and others in various stages of decay. Because of the high oil content of this particular species of cypress, they decompose very slowly which means that even felled trees from centuries ago were still intact on the forest floor. They appear in good health because other trees and plants have piggy-backed their way on to them and sometimes it is difficult to tell where one tree ends and the other begins.

It is this outward appearance that all is well that rings true with these trees and us. Like the great sugi trees, we can appear just fine on the outside while the rest of us is busy gradually decaying. Many imbalances occur gradually in the body over a long time and if you do not seek to redress the imbalance, then just like the tree, symptoms may take their time but will eventually appear.

Sha often comes to the skin without any symptoms in that particular area. Internal imbalance gradually develops in the body and it is only when it has reached a certain stage do you see the signs and feel the symptoms. But it is there all the same.

The action of Gua sha is affecting muscles, tendons, channels and points all of which can help prevent imbalance and illness. Petechiae, while seen as beneficial, does not have to appear to feel the long-term benefit or prevent ill-health.

A maintenance routine when done regularly, and in conjunction with an appropriate diet and lifestyle, can help maintain good health.

You could follow a combination of any of the sequences in this book providing of course that the treatment lasts no longer than thirty minutes. Start at the top and work your way down selecting the sequences that feel comfortable.

- Head
- Face
- Neck and shoulders

- Arms and hands
- Chest
- Abdomen
- Back
- Buttocks, hips and legs
- Ankles and feet

There are areas however that are especially useful in guarding your health and these are located in your stomach/abdominal and the mid to lower back regions. You may be familiar with the terms *yin* and *yang* and that the fine balancing act that they perform on a constant basis is how we achieve balance or imbalance in our health and wellbeing. The front of the body is thought to be yin with the Ren channel running up the midline, and the back is thought to be yang with the Du channel also on the midline. Both of these channels have a controlling function over the other yin or yang channels and contain points that can affect the very core of the body.

Regular tonifying treatment over these general areas can have a strengthening effect and so help your body in its quest for balance. They are also easily accessible areas which can be treated without any assistance. Remember that the strokes are with lighter pressure.

Do the following sequences in either order.

1. Strengthen *yin* - Abdomen sequence, especially on and near the midline.
2. Strengthen *yang* - Mid and Lower Back sequence. Including light and very cautious stroking near the Du channel on the spine. Check for any soreness between the vertebrae as this is where you can find Du points and lightly press any tender points.

With any sore or knotted areas, use a press technique.

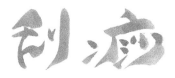

12

USE GUA SHA TO TREAT AILMENTS

HEAD AND MIND

HEADACHES

Headaches have a range of causes but are often accompanied by tension around the neck and shoulders, and over the upper back. It is usually important to remove tension in these areas as part of treating the pain in the head. Remember that although the pain is in the head, the problem does not have to be - heat can rise up, obstructions can restrict circulation and an energetic weakness can slow the body down. All of these have their roots in the body and not the head.

GENERAL AREAS
1. Head sequence (also 5 in the specific areas section)
2. Face sequence (also 3 in the specific areas section)
3. Neck and shoulders sequence (also 2 in the specific areas section)

SPECIFIC AREAS

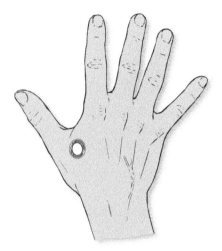

Image 74.
Large intestine 4

1. Narrow stroke and press the centre of the web between the thumb and the index finger. This is an important acupuncture point called Large intestine 4 or *Joining valley* which affects the head and the face and is often tender when pressed (image 74).

2. Narrow stroke and press a point named *Wind pool* or Gall bladder 20. This point is covered in the neck and shoulders sequence but in many cases of headaches needs further attention. It is at the base of the skull around half way between the midline and the mastoid process bone below the ear, between the sternocleido-mastoid and trapezius muscles (image 75)

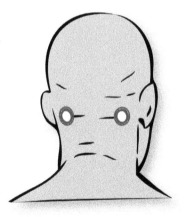

Image 75.
Gall bladder 20

3. Vibrate and press at Supreme yang or *Taiyang*. This is an important point at the temples. You can find it in the temple at the same level as the midpoint between the eye and eyebrow. Avoid heavy pressure as the temple area is sensitive (image 76).

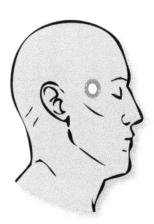

Image 76. Taiyang

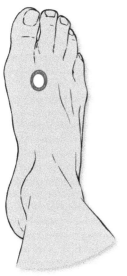

4. Narrow stroke between the first and second metatarsal bones in the foot. There is a point here called *Great rushing* or Liver 3 which has a strong effect on the body's circulation especially effective at clearing the head and eyes (image 77).

Image 77. Liver 3

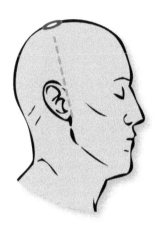

Image 78. Du 20

5. The aptly named *One hundred meetings* or Du 20 is considered to be the meeting point of all the *yang* energy in the body. It is found by following the slanted line of the ear upwards to the midline on top of the head. Wide stroke downwards from this point in multiple directions. Use short, firm strokes but light pressure (image 78).

6. Scrape down the Gall bladder channel in the upper and lower leg (image 83).

NASAL PROBLEMS

Nasal problems include hay fever, rhinitis and sinusitis. The channels that affect the nose mostly run along the arm so in addition to local treatment on the face area, the focus is on these arm channels - in particular the Lung and Large intestine channel.

GENERAL AREAS

Choose from the following sequences:
1. Face sequence
2. Head sequence
3. Arm sequence (also 1 in the specific areas section)
4. Neck and shoulders sequence

SPECIFIC AREAS

1. Wide stroke along the Lung and Large intestine channels in the arm - if *sha* appears scrape in the muscle around rather than only on the line of the channel. Remember that the *sha* does not usually follow the line of the channel (images 79 and 80).

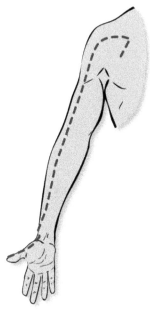 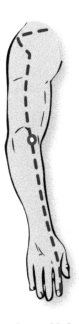

Image 79.
Lung channel

Image 80. Large
intestine channel

2. Two important Lung points are at side of pectoral muscles, where the arm meets the torso. These are the first points along the Lung channel (Lung 1 and Lung 2) and both have a direct effect on the functioning of the lungs and nose. Vibrate in a downwards or outwards direction in this area (image 81).

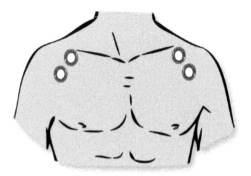

Image 81. Lung 1 & Lung 2

3. Wide stroke the area around Bladder 13 or *Lung Shu* on the upper back. This is one of the key Lung points in the body and lies half way between the vertical edge of the shoulder blade and the spine, level with the gap between the 3rd and 4th thoracic vertebrae. If the muscle around here is tight, use pressing techniques before scraping again (image 82).

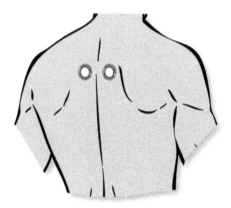

Image 82. Bladder 13

Use gua sha to treat ailments

Depression

Depression is essentially stagnation of emotions. Sometimes having the ability to go through a full range of emotions changes to being mostly stuck in just one. Treating depression is not that dissimilar to any other physical obstruction in the body. Of course there is sometimes a complex combination of factors that lie behind it, but the first step is to help the process of movement inside the body. This is where Gua sha comes in and the stagnation inside is often reflected on the surface in the form of tension in the musculature.

General areas

1. Neck and shoulder sequence
2. Mid and lower back sequence
3. Chest sequence (also 4 in the specific areas section)
4. Head sequence (also 2 in the specific areas section)
5. Foot sequence

Specific areas

1. Wide stroke along the Gall bladder channel in the lower leg (image 83).
2. Narrow stroke around Gall bladder 20 at the back of the head as described in headaches (page 139).
3. Wide or narrow stroke along the Spleen channel in the lower leg (image 84).
4. Vibrate at Lung 1 and 2 as described in Nasal problems (page 142).

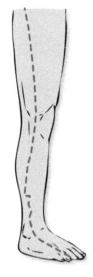

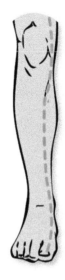

Image 83.
Gall bladder channel

Image 84.
Spleen channel

ANXIETY

There is a close connection between anxious feelings and the internal circulatory movement of *qi* and blood. Stress, work and all manner of life's trials and tribulations can lead to a tendency for either a weakness or stagnation in the chest area. In both of these cases, Gua sha can be of benefit.

GENERAL AREAS

1. Mid and lower back sequence - especially the area between the shoulder blades
2. Chest sequence
3. Arm sequence (also 1 in the specific areas section)
4. Hand sequence

Specific areas

1. Wide or narrow stroke along the Heart and Pericardium channels in the lower and upper arm (image 85).
2. Wide or narrow stroke along the Gall bladder channel in the lower leg as described in depression. Points in this area can have a profound effect on the chest (page 145).
3. Vibrate at Liver 3 as described in headaches (page 139).

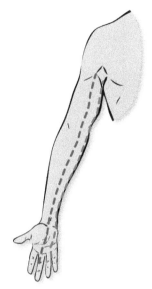

Image 85. Heart & Pericardium channel

Insomnia

For insomnia, the focus of treatment is very much on the head and neck areas as this is where many of the points associated with insomnia can traditionally be found. However like most conditions associated with the head area, treatment to the body often holds the key.

General areas

Choose from the following sequences:

1. Head sequence (also 1 in the specific areas section)
2. Neck and shoulders sequence (also 2 in the specific areas section)
3. Mid and lower back sequence
4. Foot sequence

Specific areas

1. Wide stroke down from Governing vessel 20 at the top of the head as described in headaches (page 139).

2. Narrow stroke and press at Gall bladder 20 under the occiput at the back of the head as described in headaches (page 139).
3. Wide stroke down the Du or Governing channel which runs up the centre line of the back of the body on the head and neck. Scrape cautiously and check for soreness in the gaps between the vertebrae (image 86).
4. Wide stroke along the Pericardium and Heart channels as described in anxiety. Treatment on these channels can have a deep calming effect (page 146).

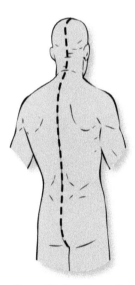

Image 86. Du channel

Dizziness

As with insomnia, an increase in the circulation of blood can help to alleviate dizziness. This is a problem that again usually stems from an imbalance in the body - either due to weakness or due to an excess of blood or *qi* rushing up to the head.

Use gua sha to treat ailments

General areas
1. Neck and shoulder sequence
2. Head sequence (also 2 & 3 in the specific areas section)
3. Hand sequence
4. Foot sequence

Specific areas
1. Wide stroke down from Du 20 at the top of the head as described in headaches (page 139).

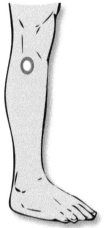

2. Narrow stroke and press at *Yang mound spring* or Gall Bladder 34 in the lower leg. This is one of the most important points in the body to remove stagnation. It can be found just below and in front of the head of the fibula bone at the top of the outside of the lower leg (image 87).

Image 87. Gall Bladder 34

3. Narrow stroke and press at a point appropriately named *Corner of the head* or Stomach 8. This has a tendency to clear the head and relieve dizziness and can be found at the top edge of the forehead roughly on a line up from the temple. This point is often tender so be cautious of how much pressure you put on the tool (image 88).

4. Wide stroke along another Stomach channel point in the lower leg called *Abundant prosperity* or Stomach 40. This is another point for clearing the head and is half way between the bottom of the knee cap and the midpoint of the lateral malleolus ankle bone. It is two finger widths from the edge of the tibia bone on the border of the tibialis anterior muscle (image 89).

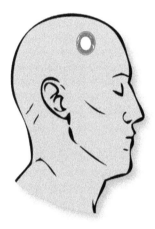

Image 88. Stomach 8

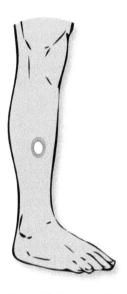

Image 89. Stomach 40

Use gua sha to treat ailments

Upper body and arms

Neck and shoulder problems

The neck and shoulder area is often where we carry the weight of our lives - our emotions, our stress, our worries - and therefore a frequent cause of discomfort, tension and stagnation. Many people are unaware of the tightness in their musculature in this area and even when they relax, or try to relax, this in-built tension remains. Try squeezing your trapezius muscle at the top of your shoulder and more often than not it feels sore often without you previously realizing it.

Problems with the shoulder joint are heavily influenced by the channels which flow over them and as these are mainly connected to the arm, this is a very useful area to treat.

Be careful with acute injuries - scraping directly on the affected area can make the condition worse. If in doubt scrape areas away from the painful one.

General areas

1. Neck and shoulder sequence (also 2 in the specific areas section)
2. Upper back sequence
3. Arm sequence (also 3 in the specific areas section)
4. Foot sequence

Specific areas

1. Narrow stroke and press the little finger side of the hand. The Small intestine channel runs in the gap between the fifth metacarpal bone and the digiti minimi muscle. As this channel runs over the upper back and neck, it has a strong influence over the neck and shoulders, especially at *Back stream* or Small intestine 3 which is to be found right below the head of the metacarpal bone, close to the base of the little finger.

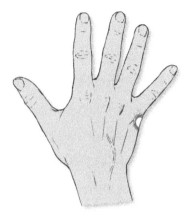

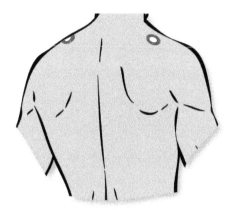

Image 90. Small intestine 3   *Image 91. Gall bladder 21*

Strokes should be short and firm and on the muscle not the bone (image 90).

2.   A local point in the neck and shoulder area which commonly presents *sha* is *Shoulder well* or Gall bladder 21 on the crest of the trapezius muscle on the shoulder, half way between the spine and the tip of the acromion. Wide stroke generally along the top of the shoulder and then short narrow stroke around this area (image 91).

3.   The arm channels have a strong influence over the neck and shoulders and certain points in particular. A point named *Outer pass* or Triple burner 6 between the ulna and radius bones, close to the wrist. Wide stroke on this point and along the Triple burner channel (image 92).

4.   Vibrate at Large intestine 4 in the hand as described in headaches (page 139).

5.   Narrow stroke around Gall bladder 20 at the back of the head as described in headaches (page 139).

6.   Narrow stroke around a point called *Narrow opening* or Stomach 38 which, despite being in the lower leg, is the main distal

point for acute shoulder pain. This can be found half way up the lower leg close to the edge of the tibia bone in the tibialis anterior muscle (image 93).

COUGHS AND BREATHING PROBLEMS

Gua sha treatment can give immediate benefits to coughs, wheezing and other respiratory problems, especially when at an acute stage. The pressure of the stroke should be stronger in acute cases and you should scrape with the intention of bringing *sha* to the surface. If *sha* does show on the skin, follow where it leads rather than having any preconceived ideas about where you believe it to be.

GENERAL AREAS

1. Upper back sequence (also 2 in the specific areas section)
2. Mid and lower back sequence
3. Chest sequence
4. Hand sequence

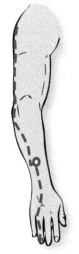

Image 92. Triple burner 6 & Triple burner channel

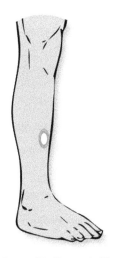

Image 93. Stomach 38

153

SPECIFIC AREAS

1. Narrow stroke around the Lung 1 and Lung 2 area at the corner of the chest as described in Nasal problems (page 142).
2. Wide stroke across a point named *Dingchuan* or *Calm Dyspnoea*. Dyspnoea is the medical term for breathlessness and this area has a specific effect on acute wheezing, cough and asthma. It can be found about one or two finger widths from the bottom of C7 vertebrae. Press if tight or tender (image 94).
3. Wide stroke along the Lung and Large intestine channels on the arm as described in nasal problems (page 142), especially over areas of soreness and tension.
4. Wide stroke along the Stomach channel in the lower leg. In particular look for tenderness at a point named *Abundant bulge* or Stomach 40 which helps to clear phlegm from the lungs and to alleviate coughing and wheezing. This point is in the tibialis anterior muscle, half way up the lower leg and about two finger widths from the edge of the tibia bone. Press if tight or tender (image 95).

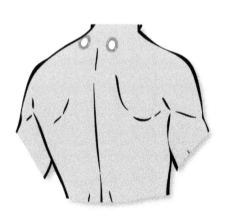

Image 94. Dingchuan

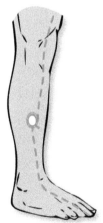

Image 95. Stomach 40 & Stomach channel

USE GUA SHA TO TREAT AILMENTS

COLDS AND FLU

This is one of the areas where Gua sha can be especially helpful. The idea behind colds and the flu is that, just as a virus might enter through the mouth or nose, so too can wind, damp, heat and cold. These natural pathogens initially can disrupt the functioning of the lungs and if not expelled in good time, will venture further in the body to cause stronger symptoms. It is best to rid the body of them as soon as possible via the pores of the skin - a process naturally done through sweating, but equally well with Gua sha. The first port of call to expel these pathogens is to use Gua sha on the neck, shoulders and upper back area.

This is a purging treatment and the focus is on removing something - in this case you want to remove the pathogens causing the disruption. You should expect *sha* to come to the surface especially in the neck, shoulder and upper back area but also in the chest.

GENERAL AREAS

1. Neck and shoulder sequence
2. Upper back sequence (also 2 & 4 in the specific areas section)
3. Chest sequence (also 1 in the specific areas section)
4. Head sequence (also 3 in the specific areas section)

SPECIFIC AREAS

1. Narrow stroke around the Lung 1 and Lung 2 area at the corner of the chest as described in Coughs and breathing problems (page 153).
2. Wide stroke around Bladder 13 on the upper back as described in nasal problems (page 142).
3. Narrow stroke around Gall bladder 20 at the back of the head as described in headaches (page 139).
4. Wide stroke along the midline from the back of the head, down the neck and into the upper back. This is following the Governing channel down the vertebrae so follow the cautions

about treating along the spine. Wide stroke also in the muscle either side of the vertebrae. An important point in this area is known as *Great hammer* or Du 14 which helps to resolve fever. It is where the neck meets the shoulders in the gap between the seventh cervical and the first thoracic vertebrae. Narrow stroke this point and those in the gaps above and below (image 96).

5. Wide stroke along the Lung and Large intestine channels on the arm as described in nasal problems (page 142).

6. Narrow stroke at Large intestine 4 in the hand as described in headaches (page 139).

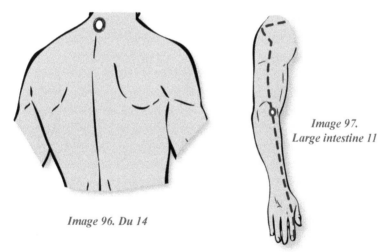

Image 97.
Large intestine 11

Image 96. Du 14

ELBOW DISCOMFORT

Lateral epicondylitis or tennis elbow is one of several sore elbow conditions that appear on or around the elbow joint. The obvious place to start with Gua sha treatment for these types of problems is with the arm sequence but be very cautious with the elbow area. If in doubt do not scrape locally, but higher up or lower down along the channels that pass over the elbow instead.

USE GUA SHA TO TREAT AILMENTS

GENERAL AREAS
1. Neck and shoulder sequence
2. Upper back sequence
3. Arm sequence (with caution in the elbow area)
4. Hand sequence

SPECIFIC AREAS
1. Narrow stroke a point called Large intestine 11 or *Crooked pond* which is found at the outside end of the elbow crease when the elbow is bent towards the body. Also wide stroke along the Large intestine channel in the arm (image 97). Avoid the elbow area in acute cases.

WRIST DISCOMFORT
The wrist is made up of small carpal bones surrounding the carpal tunnel through which tendons and the median nerve pass through and are kept in place by a thin ligament. It is very common to have pain here especially from repetitive movements like typing on a keyboard or playing racket sports.

The idea of treatment with Gua sha is to start by treating the channels that pass over the wrist but further away from the problem. The neck, upper back and shoulder area covers all these channels. Then gradually come closer with the arm and possibly the hand. Only if appropriate, would the actual wrist be treated.

GENERAL AREAS (NO SPECIFIC AREAS)
1. Neck and shoulder sequence
2. Upper back sequence (if you have assistance)
3. Arm sequence (this covers all of the arm channels)
4. Hand sequence (with caution)

Gua Sha

Lower body and legs

Lower backache & sciatica

Gua sha treatment offers many benefits to back ache and sciatica-type leg pain. These often go together as symptoms but not always, and treatment for both normally involves treating other areas away from the back area.

Be careful with acute back injuries - scraping directly on the affected area can make the condition worse. If in doubt use Gua sha in areas away from the painful area.

General areas

1. Mid and lower back sequence (with caution)
2. Buttocks, hips and leg sequence (also 1, 2 & 3 in the specific areas section)
3. Foot sequence

Specific areas

1. A local point which is often tender and requires treatment is *Jumping circle* or Gall bladder 30. This is located a third of the distance between the greater trochanter of the femur (the top of the leg bone) and the sacral hiatus (the midpoint between the buttocks). Wide stroke around this point and press any tender areas (image 98).

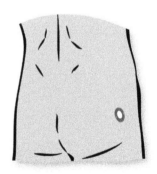

Image 98.
Gall bladder 30

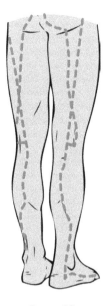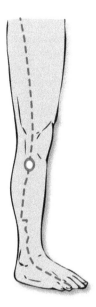

Image 99.
Bladder channel

Image 100.
Gall bladder channel

2. Wide stroke along the Bladder channel from the centre of gluteal crease (the line just below the buttocks) to the back of the knee and down towards the ankle. The Bladder channel runs through the lower back and leg area and there are several useful points both to help the lower back and to unblock the channel (image 99).

3. Another key channel for pain in the back and legs is the Gall bladder channel (image 100). Wide stroke along this channel which runs down the outside of the leg from the buttock and in particular Gall bladder 34 as described in dizziness (page 148).

Constipation

The logical place to start treatment for constipation would be the stomach and abdomen as this is the area that we associate with the intestines, but in fact it is the lower back that is often the most effective and is where you should begin. The style of treatment is more on the purging side with the expectation that *sha* will come out on to the skin, unless you feel weak or tired in which case use a gentler technique.

General areas

1. Mid and lower back sequence
2. Stomach and abdomen sequence
3. Buttock, hip and leg sequence (also 2 & 4 in the specific areas section)
4. Foot sequence

Specific areas

1. Wide stroke along the Triple burner channel in the lower arm (image 101).
2. Wide stroke along the Stomach channel in the area of Stomach 36. This is a very important point to know in Oriental medicine. This point is named *Leg three miles* because of its ability to help fatigue (hence you have the ability to walk another three miles). It can be found in the tibialis anterior muscle close to the edge of the tibia bone around 4 finger-widths below the knee. Use narrow stroking and pressing on any tender areas (image 102).
3. Wide stroke along the Large intestine channel in the lower arm, particularly close to the elbow area. Narrow stroke Large intestine 11 as described in elbow discomfort (page 156).
4. Wide stroke generally along the Spleen channel but two areas are particularly important. *Yin mound spring* or Spleen 9 is in the muscle just behind the curve of the tibia bone at the top of

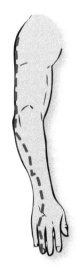
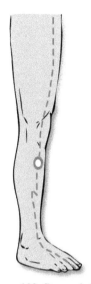
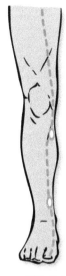

Image 101.
Triple Burner channel

Image 102. Stomach 36
& Stomach channel

Image 103. Spleen 6
& Spleen channel

the lower leg. And *Three yin meeting* or Spleen 6 is the width of four fingers above the highest point of the medial malleolus ankle bone, just behind the edge of the tibia bone. Narrow stroke the area around these points which is often sore. Use short stroke lengths and variable pressure (image 103).

DIARRHOEA

Like constipation, the place to start when treating diarrhoea is at the lower back. It too is a purging treatment to remove cold, heat or damp, although adjust the strength of treatment if you are tired and feel weak.

GENERAL AREAS
1. Mid and lower back sequence
2. Stomach and abdomen sequence (also 1 in the specific areas

section)

3. Buttock, hip and leg sequence (also 2 & 3 in the specific areas section)

4. Foot sequence

SPECIFIC AREAS

1. A local point in the abdomen called *Heavenly pivot* or Stomach 25 is often indicated in diarrhoea. It lies about three finger widths from, and level with, the belly button. Wide stroke this area but be cautious of putting too much pressure on the abdomen (image 104).

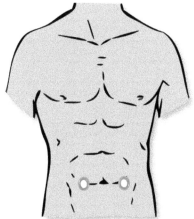

Image 104. Stomach 25

2. Wide stroke along the Stomach channel in the lower leg. In particular, narrow stroke Stomach 36 as detailed in constipation (page 160).

3. Wide stroke along the Spleen channel in the lower leg and narrow stroke and press at Spleen 9 and 6 as detailed in constipation (page 160).

STOMACH/ABDOMINAL DISCOMFORT

Stomach and abdominal pain is often caused by stagnation and increasing circulation with Gua sha will help remove this stagnation both in this area and in the body in general. As with constipation and diarrhoea, the best place to start is at the mid and lower back.

Use gua sha to treat ailments

General areas

1. Mid and lower back sequence
2. Chest sequence
3. Stomach & abdominal sequence (also 2 in the specific areas section)
4. Foot sequence

Specific areas

1. Wide stroke the midline of the inside of the lower arm along the Pericardium channel. An important point for the stomach lies three to four finger widths from the wrist in between the two central tendons. This is known as *Inner gate* or Pericardium 6 and can be narrow stroked with short stroke lengths (image 105).
2. Wide stroke around Stomach 25 on the abdomen as described in diarrhoea (page 161).
3. Wide or narrow stroke along the Stomach channel in the lower leg as described in diarrhoea (page 161).

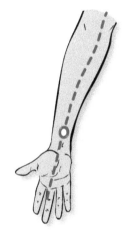

Image 105.
Pericardium channel &
Pericardium 6

Knee discomfort

The knee is a very vulnerable part of the body as it has to support the twists and turns of the body above it. Pain and discomfort can be felt from a variety of causes including tissue strain, torn ligament or tendon, tendonitis, bursitis and osteoarthritis. In terms of Oriental medicine, knee pain could be due to weakness. The knee area comes under the influence of the Kidneys and weakness of the knee is part of a wider problem of lack of energetic strength in the Kidneys. Knee pain can also be caused by stagnation or environmental factors such as damp and cold which prevent the free flow of blood and *qi*.

The knee is a bony area so most of the actual stroking action is around, not on, the knee or along channels or body parts connected to the knee.

General areas

1. Lower back sequence
2. Buttock, hip and leg sequence (also see the specific areas below)
3. Foot sequence

Specific areas

1. Wide or narrow stroke along the Stomach channel and Gall bladder channels above and below the knee (image 106). Also vibrate around Gall bladder 34 as described in dizziness (page 148).
2. Wide or narrow stroke along Spleen channel above and below the knee. Press at Spleen 6 and 9 as described in constipation (page 160).
3. Wide or narrow stroke along Bladder channel above and below the knee as described in lower backache and sciatica (page 158).
4. Press Stomach 35 or *Calf's nose* and an extra point called *Xiyan*. These points lie under the patellar either side of the central patellar ligament. Use caution with this technique if there is acute pain (image 107).

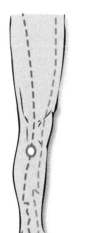

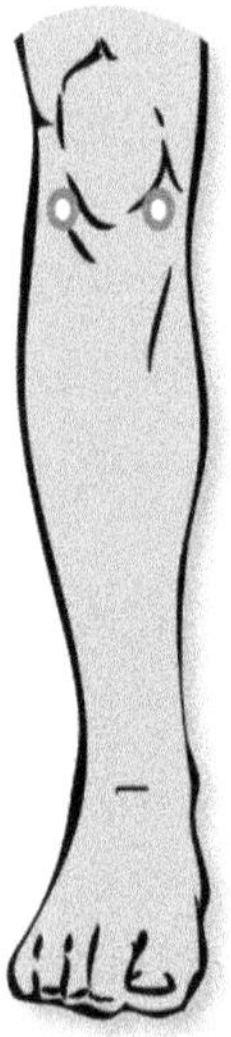

Image 106. Stomach & Gall bladder channels

*Image 107.
Stomach 35 & Xiyan*

Use gua sha to treat ailments

Ankle discomfort

The ankles are another reserve of the Kidneys both in terms of organ influence and in the actual location of the Kidney channel. Any weakness here can turn out to be an underlying weakness of the ankle joint and you can be more prone to injury and pain.

General areas

1. Lower back sequence
2. Buttocks, hips and leg sequence
3. Foot sequence (also 1 in the specific areas section)

Specific areas

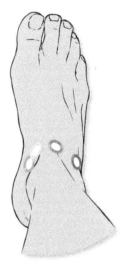

Image 108. Ankle points

1. Press local points around the extensor retinaculum sheath at the front of the ankle joint. These include points of the Stomach (yellow), Spleen (orange), Gall Bladder (dark green) and Liver (light green). The Stomach point is on the midline of the ankle joint, the Gall bladder and Spleen points are in front of and just below the bony epicondyle on their respective sides of the ankle, and the Liver point between the Spleen and Stomach channels (image 108).

Other conditions

The conditions that have been included in this section are not exhaustive and there are many more health problems that can benefit from Gua sha treatment. For treating any disorder the most important thing to remember is to look at the bigger picture, see the body as a whole and adjust the treatment according to you and your body - not just focus on a localised area or problem.

165

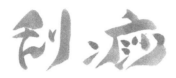

AFTERTHOUGHTS

Gua sha is part of a view of the body that sees everything connected, from the smallest molecule to the largest body part. It looks at the body holistically and sees cosmetic change as inseparable from internal change. Although Gua sha therefore has wide applications both by itself and in conjunction with other forms treatment which make it particularly useful to be used clinically, to see where its greatest potential as a preventative and curative procedure could lie, we need to look in the home.

I have lost count of the times I have treated a member of my family or them me to help combat a cold, flu, aches and pains and the symptoms of stress. Writing a book about health is ironically one of the most unhealthy things you can do. You have to glue yourself in front of a keyboard for inordinately long periods of time. My back is a testament to this and it has spectacular smudges of Gua sha induced redness not caused by any swanky Gua sha tool but by a spoon the price of a candy bar. It is not a cure-all of course but for many conditions, Gua sha is in essence is the ultimate home treatment.

One of the quirks of working here perched at the top of Africa, is that it is a rare thing to have a patient come alone. Treatment is a social thing and the patient is invariably accompanied by a relative or friend or sometimes the whole family. This is I am sure partly because of the pale skinned and heavily accented foreigner who is about to poke a loved one with an acupuncture needle the imagined size of a small javelin. I would probably want to be there too in their shoes. It is not a javelin by the way, more of a cat's whisker. They are also there out of genuine curiosity and a desire to seek out an alternative to the lopsided state of modern medicine here where drugs and surgical procedures take the place of genuine patient care.

I take advantage of these extra bodies in the room by teaching them simple things that might make a difference in the health and comfort of their relative or friend sprawled out on the treatment couch. Gua sha is often one of these techniques. I have a whole bunch of spoons sitting in the cupboard for exactly that purpose.

As with the Vietnamese who have been using Gua sha (or *Cao gio*) for many centuries, a comprehensive understanding of all the internal processes that go on is not a requirement for treatment. They only need the basics in safety and technique in order to carry out Gua sha and are unfailingly delighted to learn. Watching a loved one in pain or discomfort is a disempowering experience. There is nothing quite like the helplessness. Gua sha is one of the tools that can help to redress this. With directed home treatment the benefits run to the patient who receives the continuation of an effective treatment but also to the family member who can take an active role in relieving suffering.

The focus of this book therefore has been treatment in the home but more specifically treatment on yourself at home. This is because in order to understand the treatment, you need to experience it firsthand. You need to know how the tool feels at different angles, how hard to press on various parts of the body and when the lubricant is not enough. To understand what lies under your skin both physically and energetically and how the different parts of you are in fact connected.

We are bombarded with messages telling us how in every facet of our lives high-tech is the way to go. Cars that park themselves. TVs that work with hand gestures. Phones which are not really for calling. Even the environmental problems produced by our rampant desire for more, are to be solved by technologically tampering with anything from the weather to seeds.

Modern medicine is no different and is going at breathtaking speed - almost exclusively in one high-tech direction. As far as health goes this has meant a gradual distancing between the health provider and the patient. Tests and procedures that can be commanded by the swish of a pen or the push of a button have replaced simple human contact.

We have become accustomed to a way of living and a way of maintaining that life at all costs, including our health. Why change destructive behaviour when there is a drug or a treatment to take away the symptoms when they come. The fixation with the result and the cure is at the expense of finding and eliminating the cause which requires considerably more effort about changing how we live our lives.

Perhaps part of this is an unfortunate development of modern medicine that where there is medicine, there is profit. Huge profits. And this is where one of the issues with Gua sha lies. It is difficult to make a profit with something that can be done at little or no cost to the user. This makes it easy to ignore or to rubbish as quack medicine, despite recent research that says otherwise. It can also be controlled of course and excuses be made that you have to visit an expensive practitioner with special tools every time in order to gain the most benefit, but this is not following the history and tradition of Gua sha.

Sometimes you need to go backwards in order to go forwards. Gua sha is not a static, ancient technique but one that is adaptable and evolving and can quite happily sit amongst the medical techniques of the twenty first century. It is, in essence, as relevant now as it ever was.

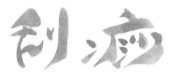

ENDNOTES

1. HUI.K, et al. 2011. Perception of Deqi by Chinese and American acupuncturists: a pilot survey. Chin Med.; 6:2.
2. BENTLEY,B. 2007. Gua Sha: Smoothly scraping out the sha. The Lantern. Volume IV, Issue 2 - Article 2. May.
3. GUILLOU,A. 2004. Medicine in Cambodia during the Pol Pot Regime (1975-1979): Foreign and Cambodian Influences. Paper prepared for the Symposium "East Asian Medicine under Communism", Graduate Center of City University of New York; July 8.
4. IMAN IBN QAYYIM AL-JAUZIYAH. 2003. Healing with the Medicine of the Prophet. Dar ul Ghad Al-Gadeed.
5. NIELSEN,A. 2002. Gua Sha: A Traditional Technique for Modern Practice. New York: Churchill Livingstone.
6. FLAWS,B. Clarifying the Meaning of Sha (as in Gua Sha) available at http://www.bluepoppy.com /blog/blogs/blog1.php/clarifying-the-meaning-of-sha-as-in-gua (Accessed 10/02/2013)
7. HAUTMAN,M.A. et al. 1987. Self-Care Responses to Respiratory Illnesses among Vietnamese. West J Nurs Res. 9: 223.
8. ZHANG XIUQIN & HAO WANSHAN. 2000. Holographic Meridian Scraping Gua Sha Therapy. Beijing: Foreign Languages Press.
9. This study on South East Asian refugees indicates that the use of 'coining' was common in at least three of the main ethnic groups studied: BUCHWALD,D. et al. 1992. Use of traditional health practices by Southeast Asian refugees in a primary care clinic. Western Journal of Medicine 06; 156(5):507-11.

10. A comprehensive review of Gua sha research can be found in NIELSEN,A. 2013. Gua Sha: A Traditional Technique for Modern Practice. Second edition. New York: Churchill Livingstone.

11. As detailed in MUDD,S & FINDLAY,J. 2004. The cutaneous manifestations of physical child abuse. J Pediatr Health Care. 18,123-129.

12. OXFORD DICTIONARIES at http://www.oxforddictionaries.com/ definition. Accessed 11th May 2013.

13. MACPHERSON Ed. 1999. Black's Medical dictionary. London: A&C Black, 39th Edition.

14. A great deal more detail can be found in the second edition of Nielson's classic Gua sha book: NIELSEN,A. 2013. Gua Sha: A Traditional Technique for Modern Practice. New York: Churchill Livingstone.

15. LANGEVIN, H.M., & YANDOW,J.A., 2002. Relationship of acupuncture points and meridians to connective tissue planes. Anat Rec. Dec 15;269 (6):257-65.

16. XINNONG, CHENG. 1990. Chinese Acupuncture and Moxibustion. Beijing: Foreign Language Press.

17. The British Acupuncture Council Guide to Safe Practice is intended for clinical practice but still has relevance here.

18. BREIVIK,H et al. 2006. Survey of chronic pain in Europe: prevalence, impact on daily life, and treatment. Eur Pain. 10, pp. 287–333

19. BENTLEY,B. 2007.Gua Sha: Smoothly scraping out the sha. The Lantern. Volume IV, Issue 2 - Article 2. May.

20. As detailed in NIELSEN, A. 2008. Gua Sha: A Clinical Overview. Chinese Medicine Times. Volume 3 Issue 4 - Winter.

21. More detail can be found in the following paper: NIELSEN,A., KLIGLER,B., &. KOLL,B. 2012. Safety protocols for Gua sha (press-stroking) and Baguan (cupping): Complementary Therapies in Medicine. 20, 340—344.

22. This arrangement is taken from the Ling Shu or 'Spiritual Axis' which is part of the ancient classic text, THE NEI JING, found in VEITH,I. 2002.The Yellow Emperor's Classic of Internal Medicine. University of California Press.

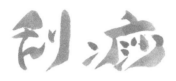

Gua sha: a complete guide to self-treatment

Clive Witham

For more information on Gua sha and Oriental medicine or
to contact the author, visit www.orientalmedicine.org

CPSIA information can be obtained
at www.ICGtesting.com
Printed in the USA
LVHW020054200419
614919LV00008B/136/P

9 780956 150738